Development of nerve cells
and their connections

Development of nerve cells and their connections

W. G. HOPKINS

Auckland University, Auckland, New Zealand

M. C. BROWN

University Laboratory of Physiology and Trinity College, Oxford, England

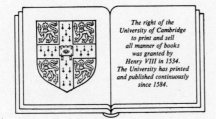

The right of the
University of Cambridge
to print and sell
all manner of books
was granted by
Henry VIII in 1534.
The University has printed
and published continuously
since 1584.

CAMBRIDGE UNIVERSITY PRESS

CAMBRIDGE

LONDON   NEW YORK   NEW ROCHELLE

MELBOURNE   SYDNEY

Published by the Press Syndicate of the University of Cambridge
The Pitt Building, Trumpington Street, Cambridge CB2 1RP
32 East 57th Street, New York, NY 10022, USA
296 Beaconsfield Parade, Middle Park, Melbourne 3206, Australia

First published 1984

Printed in Great Britain by the Garden City Press.

Library of Congress catalogue card number: 83-10097

British Library Cataloguing in Publication Data
Hopkins, W.G.
Development of nerve cells and their connections.
1. Neurophysiology   2. Cell physiology
I. Title   II. Brown, M.C.
611'.0181   QP355.2
ISBN 0 521 25344 6 hard covers
ISBN 0 521 27325 0 paperback

Contents

Contents

Preface

This short book gives an account of the development of the nervous system, from the early embryonic stages when nerve cells first appear through to the adult, where interactions between nerve cells are the basis of learning, memory and recovery from injury. Vertebrates and invertebrates are considered.

The book is intended to be used both as a text for undergraduates and graduates, and as a source book for those teaching courses on neuronal development. Scientists who wish to fill in gaps in their knowledge of this rapidly expanding field should also find this book particularly useful. Key references are provided for those wanting to read in greater detail about the issues discussed. We have assumed that readers have an elementary knowledge of basic neurophysiology and neuroanatomy.

Acknowledgements

We should like to thank Drs H.F. Brown and D.C. Van Essen and Miss Christine Booth for critically reading early drafts of this book and providing useful suggestions. Drs M.R. Bennett, J. Fawcett, M. Ito, M. Jacobson, F.A. Miles, V.H. Perry, J. Scholes and P.D. Wall very kindly provided oral or written advice on a variety of topics. We should also like to thank Miss Christine Lake and Miss Debra Allen for typing. Part of the book was written while one of us (M.C.B.) was on sabbatical leave at the California Institute of Technology. W.G.H. was supported by the New Zealand Medical Research Council.

PART I
Introduction

The nervous system is arguably the most complex structure known to man, and certainly the most complex organ system in the body. The complexity of the nervous system is due in part to its large number of cells (about 10^{12} neurons in man and at least as many glial cells), and in part to its large number of different kinds of cell (probably several hundreds or possibly even thousands). In both these respects other organ systems can be compared with the nervous system: for example, there are as many cells in the digestive system, and at least as many different kinds of cell in the immune system. However, the nervous system differs from any other part of the body in that neurons make precise patterns of connections onto other neurons, and it is this unique property that generates the complexity of the nervous system and the diversity of its actions.

The development of the nervous system is a remarkably complex process and not surprisingly many features of it are still mysterious. In recent years an increasingly large number of scientists have become involved with research on developmental neurobiology, and it is probable that newly developed techniques will solve many of the problems that have daunted previous generations of neurobiologists. Investigation of neuronal development, as is the case in most other fields, is carried out both because of the intrinsic curiosity of those concerned and because a better understanding of the mechanisms involved will have benefits for man. Abnormalities arising in development and as a result of disease or accident later in life may be alleviated by application of the new knowledge, and a better understanding of brain development will probably provide a better understanding of normal brain function. Indeed, normal function and the development of a normal brain are intimately linked processes, as will be shown in part IV.

In the following introductory chapter there is a very brief outline of the normal sequence of events in brain development and then the methods and the design of experiments used in research in this field are given.

I.1

A short outline of neuronal development

In the vertebrate the cells whose descendants contribute predominantly to nervous tissue are first identified as the neural ectoderm, a disc-shaped part of the ectoderm on the surface of the sphere of embryonic cells. This disc elongates and rounds up to form a tube within the ectoderm. Further regional elongation, outpocketing, folding and thickening of this tube produces the gross anatomical divisions of the central nervous system. At the time of closure of the neural tube some cells break away to form a transient structure called the neural crest. The cells of the crest migrate away from the neural tube and form the ganglia of the peripheral nervous system. The fibre tracts and peripheral nerves are produced when nerve cells send out axons to their targets.

At the cellular level three major stages in brain development can be identified. These follow each other more or less consecutively, and we have made these the basis for the three main subdivisions (parts II, III and IV) of this book (see table I.1).

Part II is concerned with the origin of nerve cells. In vertebrates nerve cells proliferate in several distinct germinal areas. Post-mitotic neurons then migrate, sometimes over considerable distances, to their permanent positions. At some time near the proliferation and migration stages the nerve cells become committed to developing particular biochemical and

Table I.1. *Stages in the growth of vertebrate nerve cells*

Origin of nerve cells	Proliferation, specification and migration
Establishing connections	Axon growth, dendritic growth, synapse formation
Modifying connections	Nerve cell death, reorganisation of initial inputs, adult connectivity changes

physiological properties and connectivity patterns, i.e. their phenotype is specified.

Part III deals with the ways neurons send their axons to establish connections with one another and with peripheral targets. The tip of the growing axon forms a structure called the growth cone, which guides the axon towards its target, and which also recognises its appropriate target cells. When axons reach their target synapses form, a process involving structural and functional modification of pre- and post-synaptic membrane.

As synapses develop, a considerable proportion of nerve cells die. The connections from the remaining nerve cells are subject to extensive further remodelling as excess axon branches are removed and favourable connections are expanded and stabilised. The properties of the neuron and its target are also modified as innervation matures. Functional and structural connectivity changes can continue in the normal adult and can be induced by injury. All these modifications are considered in part IV.

The invertebrate nervous system consists of interconnected ganglia positioned usually along the midline of the animal, and also sensory neurons in the periphery. All the nerve cells develop from ectodermal cells without phases of active movement or migration. The subsequent developmental stages are similar to those of vertebrates. The results of studies on selected invertebrates (usually annelids or arthropods) are dealt with briefly where appropriate in the following chapters. For a comprehensive review of neuronal development in invertebrates see Anderson, Edwards & Palka (1980).

Background reading

Short articles and a book of collected papers giving useful overviews on developmental neurobiology are:

Anderson, H., Edwards, J.S. & Palka, J. (1980). Developmental neurobiology of invertebrates. *Annual Review of Neuroscience*, **3**, 97–139.

Cowan, W.M. (1979). The development of the brain. *Scientific American*, **241** (September), 56–69.

Hamburger, V. (1981). Historical landmarks in neurogenesis. *Trends in Neurosciences*, **4**, 151–5.

Patterson, P. & Purves, D. (1982). *Readings in Developmental Neurobiology*. Cold Spring Harbor: Cold Spring Harbor Laboratory.

I.2

Methods and techniques

Histological methods

The greatest technical problem in developmental neurobiology has always been to make neurons visible. Indeed, the science began with Ramon y Cajal's use of a nerve-specific silver stain which was discovered last century by Golgi and which is still widely used today. A short summary of methods used for identifying neurons and neuron processes in developmental studies is given below.

Silver stains. These are either of the Golgi type, which stain completely a small proportion of neurons, or of the reduced silver type, which stain all nerve processes with variable efficiency.

Electron microscopy. This has provided most of the knowledge about cellular structures important in cell migration, axon growth, synaptogenesis and remodelling of connections. Many of the methods devised for identifying particular neurons in the light microscope have been adapted to the electron microscope, although many questions remain to be answered at the level of light microscopy.

Histochemistry. Some neurons can be visualised by means of their transmitter or transmitter enzymes. Catecholamines fluoresce in ultraviolet light in formaldehyde-fixed tissue, and this has been very useful in assaying the presence of adrenergic neurons. Cholinergic neurons can be detected by the presence of accompanying acetylcholinesterase.

Immunohistochemistry. Sera, or monoclonal antibodies specific for particular cell antigens, are bound to tissues and then revealed 'indirectly' by binding anti-antibodies coupled with horseradish peroxidase or fluorescent markers.

Horseradish peroxidase (HRP). This enzyme is transported within cells, both towards and away from the cell body. It can be injected or cells will take it up spontaneously. It is used to trace pathways or identify cell bodies when fixed sections of tissue are incubated with appropriate substrate. HRP is also retained in the descendants of dividing cells and can be used to identify clones.

Fluorescent markers. These are used like HRP but are visualised with ultraviolet microscopy. Other dyes and substances such as cobalt have also been used to trace axons.

Autoradiographic tracing. Radioactive substances are transported along nerves in the same way as HRP, and are visualised by autoradiography of sectioned material. In some cases the labelled material crosses synapses and delineates further pathways (transneuronal autoradiography).

Chimeras. Embryonic neural cells (and their descendants) from one species transplanted to another are subsequently identified in the chimera through interspecies differences in histology of cells, e.g. structure of the nucleolus. Cells transplanted from an animal of the same species can be identified in a chimera if they are prelabelled with an intracellular marker, such as HRP.

Birth-dating of neurons. A pulse of tritiated thymidine is incorporated into the DNA of the dividing precursors of nerve and glial cells and detected in these cells or their descendants by autoradiography.

Physiological methods

Patterns of central connections and changes in these patterns have been assayed by extracellular recording of action potentials from single cells or small clusters of cells, using wire or glass microelectrodes. Intracellular recording has been used to detect development of innervation and the changes in inputs to individual cells in the peripheral and central nervous system. Connections can also be determined by detecting biochemical changes arising as a result of activity in particular axons or pathways. In muscle, the fibres comprising a single motor unit can be identified histochemically if their glycogen levels are depleted by prior activation. Neurons can be identified by a non-metabolisable glucose analogue (2-deoxyglucose) which accumulates in active cells and can be detected autoradiographically.

Biochemical methods

Levels of transmitter and transmitter enzymes in some tissues have been used to determine changes in innervation. Effects of innervation or denervation on transmitter metabolism and RNA and protein synthesis in the nerve cell bodies have also been monitored in this way.

Experimental design

Armed with technical expertise, what kinds of experiment can the developmental neurobiologists do? There are three basic designs.

1. *Description of events in the normal animal.* The first stage in any study is to observe to the limit of the techniques available what happens in the normal developing animal. Such phenomenological observations give clues to underlying cellular and subcellular mechanisms.

2. *Description of events after experimental manipulations.* A hypothesis about mechanisms acting in the intact animal can be tested by altering conditions in an experimental animal and comparing the observed outcome with that predicted by the hypothesis. Procedures for altering conditions include either removing or translocating nerves or their targets, cutting or crushing axons and allowing them to regenerate, and changing the level of substances (e.g. hormones, transmitters, growth factors) thought to be important for an observed developmental phenomenon.

Observations on development in animals with single gene mutations affecting the central nervous system also belong to this category of experimental design. One of the drawbacks with these mutants is that a mutation in a single gene may affect several kinds of cell and several closely related developmental events, and this makes it difficult to disentangle causes and effects of the observed defects.

3. *Analysis of events in tissues* in vitro. The study of development in organ or tissue culture offers the possibility of testing a hypothesis by altering conditions in ways which are not practical *in vivo*. Conditions in culture are sufficiently different from those in the animal to leave a doubt about the relevance of events seen in culture to those that occur in the animal. Notwithstanding this doubt, the culture approach has been particularly valuable in demonstrating the importance of chemical factors in guiding neuron growth and in keeping neurons alive. It has also been useful in determining some of the mechanisms of synaptogenesis and neuronal differentiation. The chick embryo chorioallantoic membrane is an organ culture environment more closely approximating that of the whole animal, and has been used to study the development of neurons of the peripheral nervous system.

Most publications report the results of work on a single animal species, chosen from considerations of economy, availability and ease of experimentation for the particular developmental phenomenon being studied. Generally the findings should not be assumed to apply more widely until they are confirmed in other species.

PART II

Genesis of nerve cells

Synopsis

In invertebrate species it has been possible to follow the development of specific, identified neurons from earlier precursor cells. These studies have revealed stereotyped patterns (lineages) of cell division and cell differentiation, suggesting that the characteristics (phenotypes) of particular neurons are determined at the time of mitosis of precursor cells by asymmetrical cell division. Some neuronal phenotypes in invertebrates are also determined by the action of local environmental signals on uncommitted precursor cells, a process known as induction. The signals that determine phenotypes in either lineage or inductive specification have not yet been identified.

In vertebrates commitment of embryonic cells to neuronal development has long been thought to begin at the gastrula stage when mesoderm, migrating under the ectoderm, induces it to become neural ectoderm. However, it has been claimed recently that this classical theory of primary neuronal induction is incorrect and that specification of the major subdivisions of the nervous system may begin at the 512-cell blastula stage.

Little is known about the origins of the specific nerve cell phenotypes in the vertebrate central nervous system, but investigations of the origins of the peripheral nervous system have been more successful. Peripheral neurons are derived from the neural crest, a transient aggregate of cells that detaches from the edge of the neural ectoderm at the time of closure of the neural tube. The crest cells migrate out into the periphery, where specific phenotypes are induced by local influences.

Proliferation of nerve cells after neural tube closure occurs only along the inner surface of the neural tube, and later at a few sites on the outer surface of the brain. Post-mitotic neurons migrate radially through adjoining tissues to their characteristic locations. The migration appears to be guided by radially oriented glial cell processes. Migration of neural crest cells and the tangential migration of neurons of the central nervous system to secondary proliferative zones occur along specific pathways with surface properties that are different from those of surrounding tissues. Migration may be controlled by the expression of differential cell affinities on the cell surfaces.

II.1

Origin and differentiation of nerve cell types

In any one region of the nervous system there are usually distinct sets of neurons that differ in their morphologies, patterns of connections, transmitter synthesis and transmitter sensitivities. Cells of a given set can also carry distinct surface labels that allow the ordered patterns of connections between one region and another to be established. All these distinguishing characteristics taken together are called the phenotype of a neuron. Altogether there are probably hundreds of distinct nerve cell phenotypes in an individual animal.

All these phenotypes have to be generated from uncommitted, dividing precursor cells, and there are in principle only two distinct mechanisms that can achieve this (fig. II.1). In *lineage* (or intrinsic) *specification*, an asymmetric cell division distributes some sort of cytoplasmic determinant unequally between the daughter cells and thereby confers different fates on

Fig. II.1. Two mechanisms for specification of phenotype.

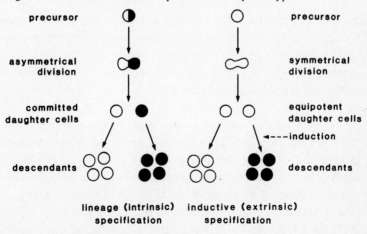

precursor / asymmetrical division / committed daughter cells / descendants — lineage (intrinsic) specification

precursor / symmetrical division / equipotent daughter cells / ◄---induction / descendants — inductive (extrinsic) specification distinct daughter cells and their descendants. In *inductive* (or extrinsic) *specification*, different fates are conferred on identical daughter cells by a position-dependent, inductive signal. To determine the nature of the mechanism that specifies particular phenotypes, the precursors of these phenotypes first have to be identified in the embryo, and then an appropriate experiment on the precursors has to be devised. The precursors are identified and their fates traced by means of a cell-marking or vital-staining technique, or by direct observation if this is possible. Subsequent experiments include killing or removing some precursors, changing their position in the embryo, or changing their surrounding environment. If the fates of precursors are changed by these procedures, inductive specification is strongly indicated, and some clue to the nature of the inducing signal can be inferred by comparing the environments that induce different fates in the precursors. Unchanged fates mean either that specification is intrinsic or that fates have been determined before the experimental intervention.

In invertebrates neuronal phenotype appears to be specified mainly by lineage mechanisms that utilise invariant patterns of cell division, with the environment inducing only some characteristics. Specification of the precursor cells that will give rise to the vertebrate nervous system appears to be inductive, although this may occur at an earlier stage and by a different mechanism than has been generally accepted. Little is known about the subsequent specification of specific nerve cell phenotypes in the central nervous system, but in the peripheral nervous system it has been shown that the transmitter phenotypes expressed by descendants of the neural crest are probably determined by local environmental influences.

Specification in invertebrates

The small number of cells in invertebrates and their accessibility for observation and manipulation make it possible in some cases to identify specific individual neurons in the adult and in the embryo and to construct detailed lineages linking these cells. This has been achieved with the nematode, leech and grasshopper.

Nematode. In the adult nematode worm, *Caenorhabditis elegans*, there are less than 1000 cells, and of these only 300 are neurons. Direct observation of living cells using Nomarski optics in combination with analysis of serial electron micrographs has led to the identification of every cell in the animal in the post-hatching stages of development, and has revealed stereotyped, invariant patterns of cell division and differentiation (Sulston & Horvitz, 1977). For example, neurons of the ventral cord are generated by a stereotyped set of divisions of 12 precursors (P cells) aligned along the anterior–posterior axis of the animal (fig. II.2). The daughter cells of a given P cell are all quite different in their phenotypes, but the daughter cells that arise by the same branch in each of the 12 lineages (lineally equivalent progeny) have similar phenotypes. These patterns of cell division and differentiation are easily explained by lineage specification but with difficulty by any inductive mechanism. Further investigation of the specification mechanism has been carried out by reconstructing lineages either in normal animals in which identified precursors have been killed with a laser microbeam, or in mutants with lineage abnormalities. Fates of surviving daughter cells are usually unchanged in these animals, even though they or their progeny occupy abnormal positions (Sulston & White, 1980). However, there are instances in the normal animal where a precursor can go through either of two lineages, and the choice appears to depend on its position in the animal. Moreover not all lineally equivalent progeny have the same phenotype: for example, the cells of the P.aap subset that are distant from the gonad die, and those of the hypodermal subset that are in contact with the gonad undergo further divisions (Sulston & Horvitz, 1977). This makes it likely that induction, in this case possibly an influence

Fig. II.2. Above: nematode immediately after hatching, showing positions of the 12 P precursors of the ventral cord. Below: typical lineage of descendants of each P cell (a, anterior; p, posterior).

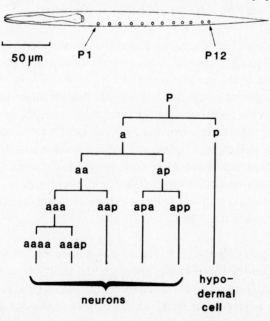

from the gonad, can contribute to determination of phenotype in the nematode.

Leech. The longitudinal axis of the leech is established when a number of the large ectodermal cells (teloblasts) in the early embryo bud off long lines of cells (germinal bands). Fluorescent dye coupled to a protein injected into the teloblasts is retained in their progeny in the germinal bands and in the developing segmental ganglia, making it possible to show that four identifiable teloblasts give rise to all but one of the ganglia of the nervous system. Injection of a single teloblast reproducibly stains a unique set of cells in each of the segmental ganglia, so it is likely that specific neurons in the ganglia are invariably descended from specific teloblasts. To determine whether specification is by lineage or by induction, so far only the effect on the development of the ganglia of teloblast ablation, achieved by injection of proteases, has been investigated. Destruction of the teloblast that provides most of the neurons in the ganglia leads in many cases to the total absence of neurons in the half-ganglia on the ablated side, even though the other teloblasts providing neurons to the ganglia were initially unaffected. Destruction of the teloblast giving rise to the mesoderm also results in the absence of half-ganglia on the affected side (Stent & Weisblat, 1981). These experiments demonstrate that environmental influences are likely to be important in ganglion formation, but it is not yet clear whether these influences permit the expression of phenotypes already determined by lineage, or whether there is a true induction of phenotypes.

Grasshopper. The nervous system in the grasshopper is a series of paired, segmental ganglia that arise from a longitudinal strip of ectodermal cells. The neurons of the ganglia arise from two types of large neuronal precursor cell in this strip: neuroblasts and midline precursor cells. The pattern and number of these cells is virtually constant in each body segment at the site of each future ganglion, and cell divisions that give rise to the neurons are also stereotyped. There are, however, segment-specific differences in the final expression of phenotype, in that neurons in some ganglia die, while others have quite different morphologies in different ganglia, so a combination of intrinsic and extrinsic specification probably occurs (Goodman & Bate, 1981).

Metamorphosing insects. In insects which undergo a major metamorphosis between the larval and adult stages the adult nervous system arises neither completely anew nor by unaltered adoption of the larval one. Certain neurons do persist but resorb old branches and develop new ones

(Truman & Reiss, 1976), and neuroblasts retained within the larval nervous system generate many new cells (Edwards, 1977). New sensory neurons develop from the imaginal discs, which are small groups of embryonic cells that proliferate during metamorphosis and give rise to cuticle, wings, antennae and other structures. The descendants of the cells of the imaginal discs remain within certain regions or 'compartments' with well-defined boundaries, but precisely how the sensory neurons and other cell phenotypes within each compartment are specified is not yet clear (see for example Morata & Lawrence, 1977).

Primary neuronal induction in vertebrates

There is debate about the timing and mechanism of neural specification in vertebrates. The classical picture, derived from the work of Spemann (1938), is that mesoderm lying beneath the dorsal ectoderm induces neural properties in it at the gastrula stage of development (fig. II.3). The mesoderm itself is thought to acquire its 'neuralising' capacity as it passes the dorsal lip of the blastopore (the so-called organiser) during gastrulation. The evidence for this scheme came from transplantation experiments in amphibian embryos. Transplantation of the blastopore region to another region of a host embryo could cause the development of a whole new nervous system from host ectoderm; mesoderm transplanted into a host embryo could, even when it was sited beneath ventral ectoderm (which does not normally give rise to nervous tissue), induce a second neural tube to form; and lastly dorsal ectoderm transplanted to a host could give rise to a second neural tube only if the ectoderm was taken after mesoderm had migrated in under it (i.e. after gastrulation).

The nature of the signal passed to the mesoderm and that passed from mesoderm to ectoderm to induce the ectoderm to form neural tissue has remained elusive. After many years of research, including studies *in vitro* in which mixtures of ectoderm, mesoderm, cell extracts and a variety of

Fig. II.3. Development of neural ectoderm (dashed lines show planes of section).

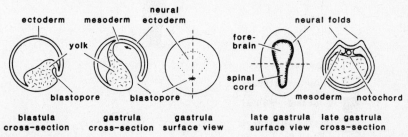

chemicals have been tested, the consensus appears to be that induction of neural ectoderm is mediated by diffusible agents from the mesoderm (Saxén, 1980), and that differentiation into forebrain, hindbrain and spinal cord may depend upon the length of time ectoderm is in contact with these agents.

More recently, doubt has been cast on Spemann's observations and hypotheses by Marcus Jacobson, on the basis of his work with a new technique for tracing the fates of the descendants of cells of the blastula. In this technique individual cells in blastulae up to the 1024-cell stage are injected with horseradish peroxidase (HRP) and their descendants detected histochemically in sections of the embryo at later stages of development. By injecting particular blastomeres of early blastulae, Jacobson can reproducibly label restricted regions of the nervous system in later embryos. If the labelled precursor cells of these restricted regions are transplanted at the late blastula stage (i.e. before gastrulation) into another late blastula in a variety of locations, then the cells divide, migrate into the developing nervous system of the host, and assume the same morphology and positions that they would have assumed in the original donor embryo. This seems to indicate that cells are irreversibly specified to contribute to neural tissue already in the blastula, and not as Spemann hypothesised after

Fig. II.4. Compartments in the central nervous system at the time of their appearance (left) and just before formation of the neural tube (right). Cells apparently intermingle within but do not cross compartment boundaries. (After Jacobson, 1980.)

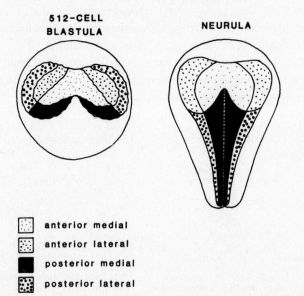

512-CELL
BLASTULA   NEURULA

☐ anterior medial
☐ anterior lateral
■ posterior medial
▨ posterior lateral

gastrulation (Jacobson, 1982). The considerable cell movements that have been revealed by HRP in this type of experiment might also explain some of Spemann's results, if Jacobson is correct.

A specification event may occur at the 512-cell stage, because the descendants of well-defined small groups of cells of this stage are restricted to, but dispersed within, particular well-defined regions of the nervous system that are analogous to the compartments derived from insect imaginal discs (Jacobson, 1980) (fig. II.4). The cells are probably restricted to their compartments by surface properties which produce selective affinities between cells of a compartment. However, the significance of the compartments and the mechanism by which they are set up remain to be elucidated.

Specification of phenotypes in the vertebrate central nervous system

In the central nervous system very little is known about the mechanisms whereby individual nerve cell types are specified, but the method of injecting HRP into single cells in the embryo will probably lead to descriptions of vertebrate cell lineages as detailed as those of in-vertebrates. Thus it has proved possible to identify the blastomeres in very early blastulae that give rise to Rohon-Beard cells (large, primitive sensory neurons in the spinal cord and the first neurons to become post-mitotic: Jacobson, 1981a). Destruction of one of these blastomeres at the 16-cell stage causes generation of Rohon-Beard neurons from adjacent blasto-meres that do not normally contribute to the Rohon-Beard population (Jacobson, 1981b). This observation is consistent with specification by induction rather than by a lineage mechanism. The timing and position of the specification event for Rohon-Beard cells may give some clue to the nature of the specification mechanism for these cells.

Another aspect of neuronal phenotype that has been studied recently is the development of neuron-specific membrane properties. Cells of the vertebrate neural plate *in vivo* and *in vitro* develop action potentials dependent first on calcium and then on sodium ions, and then become sensitive to neurotransmitter. If ways can be found to alter the develop-ment of these properties then this system may yield information on the specification mechanism. This work has also shown that cells are coupled by low-resistance junctions around the time specification of some neurons occurs, and it may be a useful approach to determine whether such coupling is involved in phenotype specification (Spitzer, 1981).

One further promising approach for studying cell lineages in vertebrates involves the use of histochemical techniques to detect cell-type-specific markers which are expressed by cells as they differentiate. Antibodies to a glial-specific protein bind to a subpopulation of the dividing cells in the ventricular germinal zone of the mammalian forebrain, which suggests that glial and neuronal precursors co-exist within the embryonic proliferative zones and that glia begin to differentiate well before the last cell division (Levitt, Cooper & Rakic, 1981). Other markers which distinguish different types of glial cell are also being examined (Abney, Bartlett & Raff, 1981).

Derivatives of the neural crest

The neural crest forms as a transient structure when cells detach from the edge of the neural ectoderm at the time of closure of the neural tube. The cells migrate out into the periphery and differentiate into all of the neurons and glia (Schwann cells) of the peripheral nervous system, as well as mesenchymal tissues in the head and melanocytes in the skin.

In contrast to the uncertainty about specification of central neurons, considerable progress has been made in understanding how the peripheral nervous system arises from the neural crest. A major contribution has come from Le Douarin and her colleagues, who have used the so-called xenoplastic grafting method for establishing lineages (Le Douarin, Smith & Le Lièvre, 1981). In this technique tissues from quail embryos, the cells of which contain a prominent nucleolus, are transplanted to chick embryos. The resulting chimeras develop normally and the graft and host cells or their descendants are readily distinguished in the light or electron microscope. Experiments in which small amounts of crest are transplanted to embryos of the same age and to the same level of the crest (isochronic and isotopic grafts) show that particular ganglia and nerve plexuses in the peripheral nervous system arise from particular levels of the crest. Moreover, each level of the crest gives rise to several phenotypes; for example crest from somite levels 18–24 gives rise to adrenomedullary cells as well as sympathetic and sensory ganglia and melanocytes (fig. II.5).

These observations lead to the important question of whether the different phenotypes are specified before, during or after the migration of the crest cells. One way to investigate this question is to see whether crest transplanted from one level to another behaves according to its level of origin or according to its grafted level. It has been found that the crest cells usually behave exactly like the crest they replace. For example, crest migrating from the level of somites 1–7 does not contribute to any sympathetic ganglia but instead invades the gut, where it expresses parasympathetic phenotype (detected by the presence of acetylcholinesterase). When crest from this level was transplanted to the region of somites 18–24 the cells migrated to the future sites of the sympathetic ganglia and adrenal medulla and developed adrenergic phenotype (detected by catecholamine fluorescence) but not cholinergic phenotype (Le Douarin & Teillet, 1974). This indicates that it is either the pathway or the destination, but not the original level of the crest, that is important in determining phenotype.

A different sort of experiment was then performed to show that the migration pathway itself does not determine phenotype. Crest cells from a level that does not normally give rise to cholinergic phenotype and does not colonise the gut were transplanted directly into a segment of aneural gut. This was then cultured on the chorioallantoic membrane to ensure that no other crest cells could migrate into it. The implanted cells developed high activities of acetylcholine-synthesising enzyme and cholinesterase, showing that some influence from the gut tissue was inducing the cholinergic phenotype (Smith, Cochard & Le Douarin, 1977). Moreover, strong catecholamine fluorescence was induced if a segment of the notochord was also implanted into the gut, suggesting that the notochord, which lies alongside the developing sympathetic chain, is one source of an adrenergic inducing signal (Teillet, Cochard & Le Douarin, 1978).

The simplest explanation for the results of these experiments is that transmitter phenotypes can be induced in uncommitted crest cells by local influences in the periphery. There are some indications, however, that the crest may not be a completely uniform population of uncommitted cells. In the experiment in which crest was implanted into the gut, melanocytes developed in the gut wall, suggesting that they are specified before migration. Similarly crest from cephalic levels contributes to mesenchymal tissues while trunk crest does not, but cephalic crest grafted to the trunk still gives rise to mesenchyme, suggesting that the mesenchymal phenotype is

Fig. II.5. Formation and migration of the neural crest at the level of somites 18–24, producing dorsal root ganglia (DRG), sympathetic ganglia (SG), adrenomedullary cells (AM) and melanocytes (M).

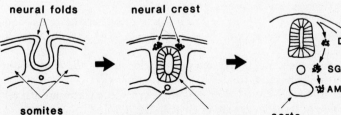
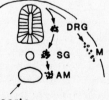

neural folds   neural crest

somites
(mesoderm)   notochord   neural tube   aorta

prespecified in cephalic crest. Thus local environmental influences may operate to some extent by selecting the appropriate crest cells from a heterogeneous, prespecified population, either by promoting the survival of particular cells at a final destination, or by diverting or inhibiting their migration.

Transplants of various developing ganglia back into younger embryos (heterochronic and heterotopic transplants) have provided evidence that developing sensory neurons can be respecified to become autonomic neurons. Moreover glia appear to be able to redifferentiate to produce neurons, which suggests that an as yet unknown inductive influence produces glia and neurons from common precursors in the crest population (Le Lièvre *et al.*, 1980).

A later stage in the development of the sympatho-adrenal derivatives of the crest is being investigated by Patterson and his colleagues (see Landis & Patterson, 1981). In their experiments sympathetic ganglia from newborn rats are cultured under different conditions to determine how a small but significant fraction of the ganglion cells becomes cholinergic while the remainder become adrenergic. It has been found that culture medium conditioned by certain non-neuronal cells from ganglia or other tissues (e.g. heart muscle) stimulates cholinergicity in the ganglion cell cultures, whereas electrical activity or depolarisation favours adrenergicity (Patterson & Chun, 1977; see also Patterson, Potter & Furshpan, 1978). This suggests that activity patterns imposed by different presynaptic connections, agents released in the ganglion, and agents released by post-synaptic targets could all be important inductive influences *in vivo*. Further support for the importance of local chemical influences is provided by the observation that the adrenomedullary phenotype is enhanced *in vitro* by glucocorticoids, mimicking the presumed influence of the adrenal cortex *in vivo* (Landis & Patterson, 1981). Attempts to isolate the possible chemical inducers are now being made (Weber, 1981).

References

Specification in invertebrates

Edwards, J.S. (1977). One organism, several brains: evolution and development of the insect central nervous system. *Annals of the New York Academy of Sciences*, **299**, 59–71.

Goodman, C.S. & Bate, M. (1981). Neuronal development of the grasshopper. *Trends in Neurosciences*, **4**, 163–9.

Morata, G. & Lawrence, P.A. (1977). Homoeotic genes, compartments and cell determination in *Drosophila*. *Nature, London*, **265**, 211–16.

Stent, G.S. & Weisblat, D.A. (1981). Cell lineage in the development of the leech nervous system. *Trends in Neurosciences*, **4**, 251–5.

Sulston, J.E. & Horvitz, H.R. (1977). Post-embryonic cell lineages of the nematode, *Caenorhabditis elegans. Developmental Biology*, **56**, 110–56.

Sulston, J.E. & White, J. (1980). Regulation and cell autonomy during post-embryonic development of *Caenorhabditis elegans. Developmental Biology*, **78**, 577–97.

Truman, J.W. & Reiss, S.E. (1976). Dendritic reorganization of an identified motoneuron during metamorphosis of the tobacco hornworm moth. *Science*, **192**, 477–9.

Primary neuronal induction in vertebrates

Jacobson, M. (1980). Clones and compartments in the vertebrate central nervous system. *Trends in Neurosciences*, **3**, 3–5.

Jacobson, M. (1982). Origins of the nervous system in amphibians. In *Neuronal Development*, ed. N.C. Spitzer, pp. 45–99. New York: Plenum Press.

Saxén, L. (1980). Neural induction: past, present and future. *Current Topics in Development Biology*, **15**, 409–18.

Spemann, H. (1938). *Embryonic Development and Induction*. New Haven: Yale University Press.

Specification of phenotypes in the vertebrate central nervous system

Abney, E.R., Bartlett, P.P. & Raff, M.C. (1981). Astrocytes, ependymal cells and oligodrendrocytes develop on schedule in dissociated cell cultures of embryonic rat brain. *Developmental Biology*, **83**, 301–10.

Jacobson, M. (1981a). Rohon-Beard neurons originate from blastomeres of the 16-cell frog embryo. *Journal of Neuroscience*, **1**, 918–22.

Jacobson, M. (1981b). Rohon-Beard neurons arise from a substitute ancestral cell after removal of the cell from which they normally arise in the 16-cell frog embryo. *Journal of Neuroscience*, **1**, 923–7.

Levitt, P., Cooper, M.L. & Rakic, P. (1981). Co-existence of neuronal and glial precursor cells in the cerebral ventricular zone of the fetal monkey: an ultrastructural immunoperoxidase analysis. *Journal of Neuroscience*, **1**, 27–39.

Spitzer, N. (1981). Development of membrane properties in vertebrates. *Trends in Neurosciences*, **4**, 19–72.

Derivatives of the neural crest

Landis, S.C. & Patterson, P.H. (1981). Neural crest cell lineages. *Trends in Neurosciences*, **4**, 172–6.

Le Douarin, N.M., Smith, J. & Le Lièvre, C.S. (1981). From the neural crest to the ganglia of the peripheral nervous system. *Annual Review of Physiology*, **43**, 653–71.

Le Douarin, N.M. & Teillet, M.A. (1974). Experimental analysis of the migration and differentiation of neuroblasts of the autonomic nervous system and of neuro-ectodermal mesenchymal derivatives, using a biological cell marking technique. *Developmental Biology*, **41**, 162–84.

Le Lièvre, C.S., Schweizer, G.G., Ziller, C.M. & Le Douarin, N.M. (1980). Restriction of developmental capabilities in neural crest cell derivatives as tested by *in vivo* transplantation experiments. *Developmental Biology*, **77**, 362–78.

Patterson, P.H. & Chun, L.L.Y. (1977). The induction of acetylcholine synthesis in primary cultures of dissociated rat sympathetic neurons. *Developmental Biology*, **56**, 263–80.

Patterson, P.H., Potter, D.D. & Furshpan, E.J. (1978). The chemical differentiation of nerve cells. *Scientific American*, **239** (July), 38–47.

Smith, J., Cochard, P. & Le Douarin, N.M. (1977). Development of choline acetyltransferase and cholinesterase activities in enteric ganglia derived from presumptive adrenergic and cholinergic levels of the neural crest. *Cell Differentiation*, **6**, 199–216.

Teillet, M.A., Cochard, P. & Le Douarin, N.M. (1978). Relative roles of the mesenchymal tissues and of the complex neural tube–notochord on the expression of adrenergic metabolism in neural crest cells. *Zoon*, **6**, 115–22.

Weber, M.J. (1981). A diffusible factor responsible for the determination of cholinergic functions in cultured sympathetic neurons. *Journal of Biological Chemistry*, **256**, 3447–53.

II.2
Neuron proliferation and migration in vertebrates

It should be clear from the previous chapter that the neurons of the segmental ganglia that make up the invertebrate nervous system are generated *in situ* and do not actively migrate during development. Vertebrates, however, have adopted a very different strategy to generate the numbers of nerve cells required in a given location. In vertebrates most nerve cells in the central nervous system are born close to the ventricular surface of the neural tube and have subsequently to migrate past other cells to their final positions. Even cells generated in secondary proliferative zones have to migrate. The peripheral nervous system is also formed as a consequence of a large-scale migration of cells.

Zones of proliferation in the developing vertebrate nervous system and the movement of neurons from these zones to their final positions were first described in studies of embryonic tissue stained for conventional light microscopy. In the light microscope the early neural tube appears as a columnar epithelium in which the cells extend from the inner (ventricular) to the outer (pial) surface. Mitoses occur at the ventricular surface, and between mitoses the nuclei migrate towards the pial surface (fig. II.6). The

Fig. II.6. Migration of nuclei between mitoses and after the last mitosis in early neural tube.

pia

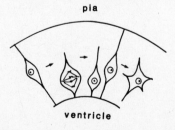

ventricle

nuclei of the first cells to become post-mitotic migrate outwards again and take up positions at well-defined levels. With the thickening of the tube the proliferating cells become localised to the inner side of the tube, thereby defining the ventricular germinal zone.

The details of the subsequent phases of proliferation and migration have been determined with the aid of tritiated thymidine (^{3}H-T) autoradiography. In this technique series of embryos and neonates are exposed to ^{3}H-T at progressively later stages of development; at a later time the animals are killed and sectioned material is subjected to autoradiography for light or electron microscopy. Neurons completing their last round of DNA synthesis at the time of exposure to ^{3}H-T are heavily labelled in all subsequent autoradiographs, while post-mitotic neurons remain free of label. The time and place of 'birth' of each type of neuron and its subsequent movement can thus be reconstructed.

Phylogenetically older neurons, for example Rohon-Beard cells, are amongst the first to be 'born' (Lamborghini, 1980). The largest neurons in any given region of the mature nervous system (e.g. pyramidal cells of cerebral cortex) are also amongst the first to become post-mitotic, apparently because they have the longest axons, and have to reach their distant targets when the embryo is still small. The smaller interneurons are generated next, followed finally by the glia, some of which continue to divide even in the mature nervous system (Lewis, 1968).

In the regions of the brain which have a laminar structure (e.g. the cerebral and cerebellar cortices) the later post-mitotic cells migrate further to the more superficial levels, so that the layers of cells are laid down in an 'inside-out' order (Angevine & Sidman, 1961). In nuclear regions (e.g. thalamus, hypothalamus) the cells accumulate in an 'outside-in' sequence (fig. II.7) (Rakic, 1977). In the mammalian forebrain a second proliferative zone, the subventricular germinal zone, develops above the ventricular germinal zone. Electron microscopic reconstructions suggest that the radial migration of post-mitotic neurons from this zone is guided by

Fig. II.7. 'Inside-out' assembly of laminar structures (left) and 'outside-in' assembly of nuclei (right).

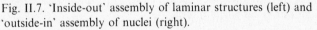
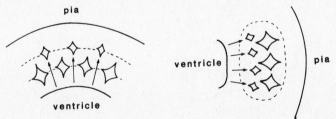

radially oriented glial cells which extend from the ventricular to the pial surface (Rakic, 1972). In the cerebellum and in the dentate gyrus of the hippocampus a germinal layer also develops at the pial surface, when dividing cells detach from nearby proliferative regions and migrate laterally over and invade the adjoining outer surfaces. Post-mitotic cells from this layer in the dentate gyrus then penetrate radially to deeper layers, coming to rest in an outside(oldest)–in(youngest) sequence (Schlessinger, Cowan & Gottlieb, 1975). In the cerebellum the granule cells which arise from the external germinal layer are guided to deeper layers by glia (Bergman glial cells), and the remaining neurons are generated in an inside-out sequence (Rakic, 1971; Altman, 1972).

Regional differences in rate of cell division contribute to the production of the complex involutions and convolutions of the neural tube as the brain develops. Differences in growth rate between surface and deep cortical layers probably also contribute at a later stage of development to the formation of gyri in the cerebral cortex (Richman *et al.*, 1975), although the formation of the major sulci which are a constant feature of the adult brain may also require other unknown influences. Little is known about what determines these differences in mitotic rate and what finally limits the number of nerve cells generated in different regions of the brain, but it has been shown that different strains of mice can have consistently different neuron numbers in the hippocampus (Wimer *et al.*, 1976).

The cells of the neural crest give rise to the vertebrate peripheral nervous system when they migrate away from the neural tube and aggregate at the sites of the ganglia, plexuses and adrenal medulla (fig. II.5). The migrating cells may be guided by a tissue space of low cell density (Pratt, Larsen & Johnston, 1975) and they may also follow chemical cues (a process called chemotaxis), since the extracellular matrix along the migration pathway has a higher concentration of hyaluronate and fibronectin than has the surrounding mesenchyme (Loftberg, Ahlfors & Fallstrom, 1980; Thièry, Duband & Delouvée, 1982). Tissue spaces and chemotaxis may also guide the tangential migration of neurons in the central nervous system: for example, fibronectin is present transiently in the pathway taken by the cells that form the external granular layer in the cerebellum (Hatten, Furie & Rifkin, 1982).

Cell movements and changes in cell shape in the developing nervous system appear to be mediated at the subcellular level by microtubules and microfilaments. Microtubules may act as a cytoskeleton to produce or maintain elongation of cells or cell processes, whereas microfilaments may have a contractile role. This is inferred from the subcellular distribution of these organelles and from the selective disruptive effects of drugs such as colchicine and vinblastine, which bind to microtubule subunits, and cytochalasin B, which inhibits many cell processes involving contractile microfilaments (Karfunkel, 1974).

The migration of neurons *in vivo* may be similar to the migration of cells in tissue culture, which has been analysed in some detail. Actin- and myosin-like proteins appear to be involved, as does a specialised ruffled membrane at the leading edge of the migrating cell, but precisely how the cell moves is not yet known (Lazarides & Revel, 1979). It is also not clear how a migrating cell knows when to stop. Differential adhesion between cells is one possible mechanism, and this could also explain the aggregation of neurons into nuclei or their stratification into laminar structures. The observation that blockade with antibody fragments of a specific cell adhesion molecule disrupts histogenesis in the retina supports this idea (Buskirk *et al.*, 1980; for a review on cell adhesion in the nervous system see Gottlieb & Glaser, 1980).

References

Altman, J. (1972). Postnatal development of the cerebellar cortex of the rat. *Journal of Comparative Neurology*, **145** 353–98.

Angevine, J.B. & Sidman, B.L. (1961). Autoradiographic study of cell migration during histogenesis of cerebral cortex in the mouse. *Nature, London*, **192**, 766–8.

Buskirk, D.R., Thièry, J.-P., Rutishauser, U. & Edelman, G.M. (1980). Antibodies to a neural cell adhesion molecule disrupt histogenesis in cultured chick retina. *Nature, London*, **285**, 488–9.

Gottlieb, D.I. & Glaser, L. (1980). Cellular recognition during neural development. *Annual Review of Neuroscience*, **3**, 303–18.

Hatten, M.E., Furie, M.B. & Rifkin, D.B. (1982). Binding of developing mouse cerebellar cells to fibronectin: a possible mechanism for the formation of the external granular layer. *Journal of Neuroscience*, **2**, 1195–206.

Karfunkel, P. (1974). The mechanism of neural tube formation. *International Review of Cytology*, **38**, 245–71.

Lamborghini, J.E. (1980). Rohon-Beard cells and other large neurons in *Xenopus* embryos originate during gastrulation. *Journal of Comparative Neurology*, **189**, 323–33.

Lazarides, E. & Revel, J.-P. (1979). The molecular basis of cell movement. *Scientific American*, **240** (May), 88–100.

Lewis, P.D. (1968). Mitotic activity in the primate subependymal layer and the genesis of gliomas. *Nature, London*, **217**, 974–5.

Loftberg, J., Ahlfors, K. & Fallstrom, C. (1980). Neural crest cell migration in relation to extracellular matrix organisation in the embryonic axolotl trunk. *Developmental Biology*, **75**, 148–67.

Pratt, R.M., Larsen, M.A. & Johnston, M.C. (1975). Migration of cranial neural crest cells in a cell-free hyaluronate-rich matrix. *Developmental Biology*, **44**, 298–305.

Rakic, P. (1971). Neuron–glia relationship during granule cell migration in developing cerebellar cortex. *Journal of Comparative Neurology*, **141**, 283–312.

Rakic, P. (1972). Mode of cell migration to the superficial layers of fetal monkey neocortex. *Journal of Comparative Neurology*, **145**, 61–84.

Rakic, P. (1977). Genesis of the dorsal lateral geniculate nucleus in the rhesus monkey. *Journal of Comparative Neurology*, **176**, 23–52.

Richman, D.P., Steward, R.M., Hutchinson, H.W. & Caviness, V.S. (1975). Mechanical model of brain convolutional development. *Science*, **189**, 18–21.

Schlessinger, A.R., Cowan, W.M. & Gottlieb, D.I. (1975). An autoradiographic study of the time of origin and the pattern of granule cell migration in the dentate gyrus of the rat. *Journal of Comparative Neurology*, **159**, 149–76.

Thièry, J.-P., Duband, J.L. & Delouvée, A. (1982). Pathways and mechanisms of avian trunk neural crest migration and localisation. *Developmental Biology*, **93**, 324–43.

Wimer, R.E., Wimer, C.C., Vaughn, J.E., Barber, R.P., Balvanz, B.A. & Chernow, C.R. (1976). The genetic organization of neuron number in Ammon's horns of house mice. *Brain Research*, **118**, 219–43.

Conclusion to part II

The early stages of brain development remain, perhaps not surprisingly, the most mysterious, and the mechanisms controlling phenotypic specification, cell division and cell migration are understood only in a fragmentary way. The greatest progress has been made in the peripheral nervous system of vertebrates and in the simple nervous systems of invertebrates. In the former the control of migration and expression of phenotype of neural crest cells by environmental influences is beginning to be understood. In invertebrates, it appears that neurons may acquire some of their adult characteristics as a result of their ancestry.

PART III
Establishing connections

Synopsis

After the phases of cell division and cell migration neurons elaborate an axon and usually also dendrites in order to make and receive connections. Growth of the axon and dendrites occurs at the advancing tip of these processes, which forms a specialised structure called the growth cone. The study of growth cones in tissue culture has shown that they can be guided by contact with different surfaces and also by gradients of diffusible substances.

In the developing animal it has been found that guidance of axons occurs both by non-specific means along preformed pathways, and also by some 'active' mechanism that can direct axons arising from a particular location towards a particular part of the target area. Further refinements in establishing specific connections can then occur by means of mutual recognition between the axons and their targets. The relative importance of guidance and recognition mechanisms varies in the few model systems that have been studied during this phase of development: the orderly pattern of connections in the limb of chick embryos and in the amphibian visual system appears to be established mainly by active guidance, but specific target recognition may be important when sympathetic ganglia are first innervated, and in insect legs a series of target recognition events lays down the pattern of the peripheral nerves.

Contact between axons and their target cells results in synaptogenesis, which has been studied predominantly at the neuromuscular junction. Receptors for transmitter, having been distributed widely before innervation, become localised to the developing post-synaptic junctional membrane, while specialised release sites are induced in the presynaptic nerve terminal. Further maturation of the neuromuscular synapse does not occur unless action potentials are produced in the muscle. The peripheral branch of sensory axons takes part in the development of specialised sensory end-organs rather than synapses, but little is known about the mechanisms that underlie this.

Interactions also occur between axons and their glial cells. In peripheral nerves glial cells are stimulated to divide by initial contact with axons, but there is a subsequent myelination of larger axons and development of nodes of Ranvier. Factors which stimulate glial cell mitosis and differentiation in the peripheral and central nervous systems are being isolated.

III.1

Axon and dendrite growth

Axon growth cones

Cajal recognised that axon growth occurred at the terminal enlargement of the axon that could be seen in silver-stained preparations of embryonic tissue, and he coined the term 'cone of growth' for this structure (see Cajal, 1928, p. 363). Growth cones were observed subsequently by Harrison (1910) in the first tissue cultures to be established successfully, and later by Speidel (1942) in living tadpole tails. More recent observations have been restricted largely to the growth cones of sensory or autonomic neurons from chick or rat embryonic ganglia in tissue culture.

In the electron microscope the growth cone (fig. III.1) can be seen to contain mitochondria, vesicles, microfilaments and microtubules. Extend-

Fig. III.1. Diagrammatic representation of a growth cone. The diameters of the filopodia are enlarged by a relative factor of 10.

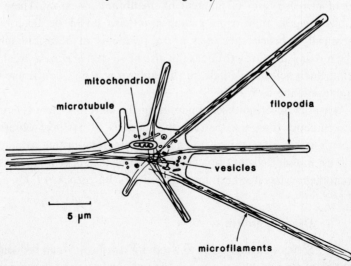

ing beyond it are fine outgrowths called filopodia (or microspikes) which are extended and withdrawn rapidly for distances of up to 50 μm. The filopodia contain microfilaments which can be stained with antibodies raised against actin, and myosin-like antigens are also present (Letourneau, 1981). Attachment of growth cones to substrates occurs mainly at points of adhesion beneath the filopodia (Letourneau, 1979), and it has been proposed that microfilaments attached at the points of adhesion pull the growth cone towards the filopodia (Letourneau, 1982). The most firmly attached filopodium would therefore be the most successful at steering the growth cone. The means by which additional membrane is added to the growth cone to enable it to advance is not certain, but a model has been proposed in which membrane vesicles are transported to the tips of the filopodia by an interaction between a myosin-like protein on the vesicle surface and the actin in the microfilaments (Bray, 1973).

There have been several clear demonstrations that growth cones grow better on surfaces to which they can adhere strongly, and that they show a graded preference for these surfaces in culture; they prefer, for example, polylysine to collagen, and collagen to agar (Letourneau, 1975). Material released from some cells, which then becomes bound to the culture dish, is also an excellent growth substrate for axons (e.g. Adler *et al.*, 1981), and this may explain why axons growing out from explants of different ganglia in culture turn selectively towards explants of their own target tissues (e.g. Ebendal & Jacobson, 1977). Growth cones will also turn towards higher concentrations of some diffusible substances, in particular Nerve Growth Factor, and there is evidence that this response is mediated by a rise in the filopodial calcium concentration (Gundersen & Barrett, 1980), which might increase rates of filament or membrane assembly. These observations suggest that axon guidance *in vivo* could be determined by chemically labelled substrates or by gradients of diffusible substances (chemotropism). Growth cones can also be steered *in vitro* by weak electric fields. Such fields could exist in the embryo and may contribute to axon guidance (Jaffe & Poo, 1979).

Attempts have also been made using the culture system to study how growth cones recognise the cells they contact. It has been observed that growth cones of sympathetic nerves form long-lasting contacts with smooth muscle cells but not fibroblasts, but the subcellular basis of this phenomenon has not been investigated (see Burnstock, 1981).

Dendrite growth

Structures analogous to axonal growth cones can be identified at the tips of developing dendrites in the light and electron microscopes (e.g.

Morest, 1969; Skoff & Hamburger, 1974). Guidance of these dendritic growth cones appears to be influenced by the surrounding tissues. A good example is provided by the dependence of cell morphologies on the parallel fibres in the cerebellum. When the interneurons in the cerebellum have their cell bodies in the middle of the parallel fibre array, they develop dendrites above and below the cell body, whereas those at the edge of the array develop dendrites only on the side of the array. Similarly in mice lacking parallel fibres the dendrites of the Purkinje cells do not develop their normal fan-like shape and are stunted (Rakic, 1975). Thus the parallel fibres appear to stimulate and direct the growth of the dendrites of these cells. The mechanism underlying the control of this growth is not known, but it probably involves contact between the parallel fibres and the filopodia of the dendritic growth cones.

Synapse formation occurs on developing dendrites and even on dendritic growth cones (Skoff & Hamburger, 1974), so synaptic input may play an important part in dendrite growth. The effects of complete block of activity on dendrite growth are not known, but a reduction in activity in the visual cortex of dark-reared animals leads to a failure in development of dendritic spines on pyramidal neurons (Valverde, 1967). Another clear example of the importance of afferent input in controlling dendritic development is seen in the Mauthner cells of fish (Kimmel, 1982), where removal of the vestibular input stunts the lateral dendrite's growth. Hormones can also influence the growth of dendrites of appropriate neurons: in a nucleus controlling song in the male canary (the singing sex) the neurons have cell bodies and dendrites that are twice the size of those in the female, but androgens can cause large neurons to develop in the female (see review by Konishi & Gurney, 1982).

For some neurons certain aspects of dendritic growth are not dependent on environmental factors but are determined by factors intrinsic to the neuron. Thus the direction of growth of dendrites of the pyramidal neurons in the cerebral cortex appears to be set by the direction of the axis of the cell body rather than by any external influences (Globus & Scheibel, 1967). Immature hippocampal neurons when dispersed in culture will develop reasonably normal primary dendritic branches (Banker & Cowan, 1979). Even the development of tertiary branches (spines) complete with post-synaptic densities can occur on Purkinje cells in the absence of the presynaptic parallel fibres (Rakic, 1975).

It is clear, then, that the overall growth of dendrites and the final shape of a given neuron is determined by a combination of intrinsic and extrinsic factors.

References

Axon growth cones

Adler, R., Manthorpe, M., Skaper, S.D. & Varon, S. (1981). Polyornithine-attached neurite promoting factors (PNPFS). Culture sources and responsive neurons. *Brain Research*, **206**, 129–44.

Bray, D. (1973). Model for membrane movements in the neural growth cone. *Nature, London*, **244**, 93–5.

Burnstock, G. (1981). Neurotransmitters and trophic factors in the autonomic nervous system. *Journal of Physiology*, **313**, 1–35 (see pp. 22–3).

Cajal, S.R. y (1928). *Degeneration and Regeneration of the Nervous System*, trans. R.M. May. London: Oxford University Press.

Ebendal, T. & Jacobson, C.-O. (1977). Tissue explants affecting extension and orientation of axons in cultured chick embryo ganglia. *Experimental Cell Research*, **105**, 379–87.

Gundersen, R.W. & Barrett, J.N. (1980). Characteristics of the turning response of dorsal root neurites towards NGF. *Journal of Cell Biology*, **87**, 546–54.

Harrison, R.G. (1910). The outgrowth of the nerve fibre as a mode of protoplasmic movement. *Journal of Experimental Zoology*, **9**, 787–846.

Jaffe, L.F. & Poo, M.-M. (1979). Neurites grow faster towards the cathode than the anode in a steady field. *Journal of Experimental Zoology*, **209**, 115–28.

Letourneau, P.C. (1975). Cell-to-substratum adhesion and guidance of axonal elongation. *Developmental Biology*, **44**, 92–101.

Letourneau, P.C. (1979). Cell–substratum adhesion of neurite growth cones, and its role in neurite elongation. *Experimental Cell Research*, **124**, 127–38.

Letourneau, P.C. (1981). Immunocytochemical evidence for colocalization in neurite growth cones of actin and myosin and their relationship to cell–substratum adhesions. *Developmental Biology*, **85**, 113–22.

Letourneau, P.C. (1982). Nerve fibre growth and its regulation by extrinsic factors. In *Neuronal Development*, ed. N.C. Spitzer, pp. 213–54. New York & London: Plenum Press.

Speidel, C.C. (1942). Studies of living nerves. VII. Growth adjustments of cutaneous terminal arborizations. *Journal of Comparative Neurology*, **76**, 57–69.

Dendrite growth

Banker, G.A. & Cowan, W.M. (1979). Further observations on hippocampal neurons in dispersed cell culture. *Journal of Comparative Neurology*, **187**, 469–94.

Globus, A. & Scheibel, A.B. (1967). Pattern and field in cortical structure: the rabbit. *Journal of Comparative Neurology*, **131**, 55–72.

Kimmel, C.B. (1982). Development of synapses on the Mauthner neuron. *Trends in Neurosciences*, **5**, 47–50.

Konishi, M. & Gurney, M.E. (1982). Sexual differentiation of brain and behaviour. *Trends in Neurosciences*, **5**, 20–3.

Morest, D.K. (1969). The growth of dendrites in the mammalian brain. *Zeitschrift für Anatomie und Entwicklungsgeschichte*, **128**, 290–317.

Rakic, P. (1975). Role of cell interaction in development of dendritic patterns. *Advances in Neurology*, **12**, 117–34.

Skoff, R.P. & Hamburger, V. (1974). Fine structure of dendritic and axonal growth cones in embryonic chick spinal cord. *Journal of Comparative Neurology*, **153**, 107–48.

Valverde, F. (1967). Apical dendritic spines of the visual cortex and light deprivation in the mouse. *Experimental Brain Research*, **3**, 337–53.

III.2

Axon guidance and target recognition

The gross patterns of peripheral nerves and nerve tracts in the central nervous system (CNS) are usually identical in different animals of the same species, so it is obvious that some form of guidance must operate when axons first grow out through their surrounding tissues. When growth cones arrive in their target area they are always confronted with at least several different cell types, so it is also obvious that some form of target recognition must exist to permit synapses to form in the long term only between appropriately matched types of cells. Closer examination of the axonal connections reveals precise point-to-point mappings connecting cells of a particular type in one region of the nervous system with their particular target cells. These ordered patterns could be established without additional active guidance or place-specific target recognition if the outgrowing axons were channelled uniformly to their target area; alternatively, labels specific to their place of origin could be carried by axons and could be used in specific guidance or recognition mechanisms.

Research on this phase of neural development has been aimed at determining unequivocally the nature of the guidance or target recognition mechanisms that operate in establishing connections in selected parts of the nervous system of various species. The experiments usually involve challenging growing axons with different tissues or targets, and then tracing the pathways taken or the connections formed. The experiments were first performed on adult animals to see whether regenerating axons would recognise selectively their former target tissues, but more recently the operations have been performed in developing animals to see whether the growth cones are guided by surrounding tissues.

In the vertebrate limb and CNS these experiments have revealed the existence of pathways that can guide axons non-specifically. In the limb, active guidance cues that direct motor axons towards their correct muscles are also present. Specific active guidance occurs in the pathway between retina and tectum in the visual system of amphibians, and while target recognition can also be demonstrated in this system in the adult, it is less clear that it is important in first establishing the correct connections. Target recognition also occurs when sympathetic ganglia are reinnervated in the adult, but it is yet to be established that the first axons reaching the developing ganglion recognise their target cells. Finally the study of the establishment of peripheral nerves in insects has revealed that a series of target cells ('stepping stones' or 'guidepost' neurons) delineate the future nerve pathways, and that the first growth cones to appear 'pioneer' the pathways between the cells in a series of target recognition steps.

Guidance pathways

Transplantation experiments designed to make axons grow through tissues they would not normally encounter have provided convincing evidence for non-specific guidance pathways in the central and peripheral nervous systems. In general the 'foreign' axons grow reproducibly along pathways which would be the sites of the normal nerve tracts in the tissue. For example, axons from transplanted embryonic retina will follow certain tracts in the developing spinal cord (Katz & Lasek, 1978), and axons from inappropriate spinal nerves will grow into transplanted limbs and produce the same gross pattern of peripheral nerves as in a normal limb (e.g. Summerbell & Stirling, 1981). It seems likely that many of the major tracts in the nervous system are non-specific, and it has been suggested that the pathways are determined in a regular geometric pattern on the neural plate (Katz, Lasek & Nauta, 1980).

Non-specific guidance could be provided by blood vessels or by boundaries between different types of tissue. Specialised structures that develop apparently for the sole purpose of axon guidance can also occur: a 'sling' of glial cells between the cerebral hemispheres plays an essential role in the formation of the corpus callosum, because the corpus callosum does not develop in mice in which the sling has been sectioned, and the sling does not develop in marsupials or mutant mice lacking a corpus callosum in the adult (Silver *et al.*, 1982). In some instances guidance can be attributed to spaces of low cell density in the tissue. For example, in the spinal cord, cell-free channels can be demonstrated between the glial cells along the sites of future tracts (Singer, Norlander & Egar, 1979). Within these channels diffusible substances released by target or other tissues may occur in concentration gradients and may exert a chemotropic influence on growth cones of specific types of nerve cell. A striking demonstration that this could be so was provided by the effects of injections of Nerve Growth Factor (NGF) into neonatal rat brains: the NGF apparently diffused down tissue spaces in the brain and spinal cord and caused a massive ingrowth of fibres from the sympathetic ganglia into the cord and up to the site of injection (Menesini-Chen, Chen & Levi-Montalcini, 1978). Substances like NGF could exist *in vivo* as freely diffusible agents or they could bind to the surfaces of the guidance channels.

Innervation of limbs

In the 1930s observations on the innervation of denervated or transplanted amphibian limbs led to the erroneous belief that specific guidance and recognition played only a minimal part in the establishment of connections between peripheral nerves and their targets. It was found that nerves regenerated into the limbs in a profuse and apparently disordered manner, and yet normal movements and reflexes were soon established. It was therefore reasoned that muscles and sensory end-organs in the limb were innervated at random, but were able to confer identity on their nerves to permit appropriate reorganisation of central connections (the theory of 'myotypic specification'). Sensory nerves innervating a piece of tadpole belly skin transplanted to the back, and back skin transplanted to the belly, were also thought to undergo a respecification of central connections to account for the misdirected reflexes which sometimes developed when the tadpoles became frogs (Miner, 1956). More recent work has shown that regenerating motor axons in salamanders and axolotls grow through the limb tissues until they find their correct muscles, even if the nerves are deliberately misdirected (Grimm, 1971), and it is likely that skin transplants in tadpoles also become innervated by their correct nerves (e.g. Heidemann, 1977). In amphibians, foreign nerves that succeed in innervating inappropriate muscles are displaced when the correct nerve returns (Dennis & Yip, 1978), but this is not the case in adult rodents (Frank *et al.*, 1975). However, in neonatal rodents a preference of regenerating motor nerves for their own muscles can be demonstrated (Gerding, Robbins & Antosiak, 1977).

These demonstrations of specific target recognition during nerve regeneration do not on their own prove that target recognition is important in establishing correct innervation during normal development. Indeed, target recognition mechanisms will not get the chance to play a part unless there is imprecision in the guidance of axons to their targets. In recent years it has proved possible to assess directly the precision of axon guidance by labelling axons with horseradish peroxidase (HRP) and then tracing and comparing the pathways of the axons in the developing and the adult animal. HRP injected into the developing muscles of tadpoles revealed that some of them are innervated by motor neurons in regions of the spinal cord that do not innervate these muscles in the adult. These erroneous projections are removed by neuronal death (Lamb, 1977; see fig. IV.3c). Thus in the frog guidance is not completely accurate and target recognition may play a significant role.

The same technique applied to chick embryos reveals, in contrast, very accurate guidance, since the motor neurons have their correct distribution in the cord from the time they can first be labelled by injections into the muscle masses (Landmesser, 1978). In the chick embryo there is a well-ordered mapping from the cord to the muscle masses from which the muscles develop: medial motor neurons project to the ventral muscle mass, lateral motor neurons to the dorsal mass, and the rostro-caudal position of neurons correlates with the axon terminations in the anterior–posterior axis of each muscle mass. This orderly arrangement could be achieved in principle by passive channelling, although it is difficult to imagine how the axons from the cell bodies of a future pool would come together passively from different spinal roots. Alternatively the identity of each pool could be specified in the cord and connections established by active guidance.

The experiments designed to determine which of these possibilities operates in the establishment of muscle innervation in chick limbs rely on observing the pattern of connections that develops when motor neurons or limbs have been translocated or partly deleted. In the most elegant of these experiments (Lance-Jones & Landmesser, 1980) a length of the neural tube consisting of three or four segments in the lumbosacral region was reversed in the cranio-caudal direction (fig. III.2). At later stages the reversed motor

Fig. III.2. Pathways taken by axons from pools for two muscles in the normal chick embryo (left). After inversion of the spinal cord axons are still guided to their correct muscles (right).

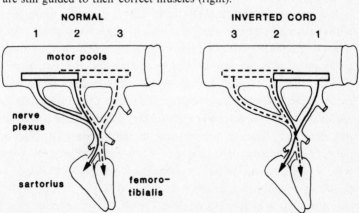

NORMAL   INVERTED CORD

1   2   3   3   2   1

motor pools

nerve
plexus

sartorius   femoro-
                   tibialis

neurons and the pathways of their axons were labelled following HRP injection into the muscles. The neurons were found to have formed their original pools and functional connections in spite of the anterior–posterior shifts in their position and axon entry point into the nerve plexus. Moreover HRP injected into specific reversed cord segments before axons had reached the muscle masses labelled the outgrowing axons in the nerve plexus and showed that they made specific alterations to their pathways to reach their appropriate muscle nerves. These observations imply that axons actively select the pathways to their own muscles by responding to local cues encountered as they grow between spinal cord and muscles.

The guidance cues are able to compensate for cord reversals and limb shifts over several segments, but axons cannot make pathway corrections for larger displacements (Lance-Jones & Landmesser, 1981) or distal limb rotations (Summerbell & Stirling, 1981). Under these circumstances non-specific cues appear to guide axons to the wrong muscles. In supernumerary limbs axons from inappropriate levels may still respond to the guidance cues in some patterned way to produce an apparent 'hierarchy of specificities' (Hollyday, 1981), but the fact that the wrong muscles are successfully innervated in these experiments is further evidence that target recognition plays a minor or negligible role in muscle innervation in chicks.

The nature and source of the specific guidance cues remain to be elucidated. Growth factors like NGF could be released by muscles to guide motor nerves, but it seems improbable *a priori* that different muscles would release different growth factors. Moreover the major axon pathways in the limb can form in the complete absence of muscle, following focal X-irradiation of somites in early embryos (Lewis *et al.*, 1981). Thus a likely role for any muscle-released factor would be to attract or stabilise the motor axons which have already been directed towards the muscles by active segmental or limb-derived cues.

The sensory innervation of chick limbs is now also being investigated with the same techniques that have been applied to the motor system. In the normal animal the initial pattern of pathways of sensory axons from the ganglia at various segmental levels is found to be the same as in the adult (Honig, 1982; Scott, 1982), suggesting the existence of an active guidance mechanism. This will be confirmed if there are specific alterations to pathways following reversal of neural crest segments, and such alterations will also prove that the sensory neuron identities are specified before the neurons reach the ganglia. Experiments are also in progress to determine whether the presence of motor axons is necessary for the establishment of sensory pathways (Landmesser & Honig, 1982).

Projection of retina to tectum

The majority of fibre tracts in the CNS connect cells in one region to cells in another in a smooth, topologically continuous manner. The establishment of order in these projections has been studied extensively in only one system: the projection of the retinal ganglion cells from the eye to the tectum, the visual processing centre in non-mammalian vertebrates (corresponding to the superior colliculus in mammals) (see fig. III.3).

Experiments on adult amphibians initiated by Sperry in the 1940s indicated that target recognition might be important in the development of the retinotectal projection. Using a behavioural assay, Sperry found that normal vision was eventually restored if the optic nerve was cut, but that inverted vision developed if the eye had also been rotated (Sperry, 1943). Sperry's explanation was that retinal and tectal cells are in some way labelled and establish their original connections on the tectum by 'chemoaffinity': following eye rotations activation of tectal regions by inappropriate parts of the visual field leads to the animal's abnormal behaviour. This view has since been substantiated by several lines of evidence. First, regenerating axons, although ultimately terminating only in appropriate circumscribed tectal locations, are disordered in the optic nerve (Fujisawa, 1981) and very widespread in their initial distribution on the tectum (Meyer, 1980). This rules out the possibility that any significant reordering occurs in the optic nerve or that regenerating axons are led straight to their original sites. Secondly, the appropriate regenerating retinal axons will make correct connections with a piece of rotated or translocated tectum (e.g. Hope, Hammond & Gaze, 1976). This implies that the restoration of a correctly oriented projection cannot be due purely to ordering of retinal axons amongst themselves on the tectal surface. Thirdly, it has been shown that cells isolated from different parts of the retina adhere preferentially to their corresponding area of the tectum (Barbera, Marchase & Roth, 1973), and a surface antigen that is expressed in a graded fashion across the retina has been identified using a monoclonal antibody (Trisler, Schneider & Nirenberg, 1981).

There is, however, a strong body of evidence showing that the labelling on the tectum does not exist as permanent markers on tectal cells. First, during normal development there is a gradual repositioning of retinal terminals on the tectum. This comes about because new retinal ganglion cells, which are added uniformly around the perimeter of the retina, project uniformly to the perimeter of the tectum, which grows only at its caudal margin (Gaze *et al.*, 1979). Secondly, when half-retinae innervate whole tecta, or whole retinae innervate half-tecta, discontinuous projections predicted by the chemoaffinity hypothesis are re-established initially, but these are gradually expanded or compressed until there is a continuous and uniform projection from retina to tectum (see review by Gaze, 1974). The new projection pattern is somehow imprinted on the tectum, since in some experiments it is re-established immediately on subsequent denervation and reinnervation (Schmidt, 1978). Moreover a normal tectum that has been denervated for six months appears to lose its labelling, because a uniform projection is established on it immediately when it is reinnervated by a half-retina (Schmidt, 1978). Thirdly, if the tectum is rotated before it is ever innervated, the subsequent retinotectal map is *not* rotated unless part of the diencephalon is also moved with the tectum (Chung & Cooke, 1978).

A number of hypotheses have to be proposed to accommodate these diverse observations (Schmidt, 1982). Positional markers must exist on retinal axons, and an interaction between fibres that maintains nearest-neighbour relationships combined with a competition for space on the tectum could explain why projections eventually become uniform. Interaction between regenerating axons and degenerating axon fragments could explain why projections appear to be imprinted initially on the tectum, or there may be some kind of transfer of label to tectal cells. Finally, the diencephalon appears somehow to provide a cue which determines the correct overall polarity for the projections.

The above discussion relates predominantly to the organisation of afferents on the tectal surface, but attention is now being focussed on the ordering of axons as they travel from the retina through the optic nerve and optic tract to the tectum. The axons from the retinal ganglion cells traverse the retina radially to the optic nerve head, and then travel down the optic nerve in a more or less orderly array (Fawcett, 1981). However, as the fibres travel through the optic tract on the surface of the diencephalon, this ordering is lost as they interweave with one another to establish a new order such that axons are delivered directly to their appropriate sites on the tectum. The reordering is demonstrated elegantly in the ribbon-shaped optic nerve and optic tract of cichlid fish (Scholes, 1979). It now seems clear that active guidance in the optic tract is responsible for this reorganisation, because the fibres that first grow out from compound eyes (produced experimentally by replacing one retinal half by its opposite half from another eye) are delivered to the tectum via the restricted branches of the tract that are appropriate for both halves of the compound eye (fig. III.3; Straznicky, Gaze & Keating, 1981). This active guidance is probably expressed on the surface of the diencephalon, and may explain the polarising ability of the diencephalon in the experiments of Chung &

Cooke, since in their animals the axons enter the tectum at the site of the repositioned diencephalon.

An intriguing problem of guidance in the CNS is exemplified by the retinotectal projection at the optic chiasm. Here the bundles of axons of identical type and function from each eye pass through each other (decussate) as they run to their contralateral termination sites. Many similar projections occur throughout the sensory and motor systems. The simplest and possibly the only plausible explanation for the phenomenon of decussation is that axons tend to grow in straight lines, and because they converge at approximately 90° in the region of decussation they cross into the contralateral pathway. The problem is particularly vexatious at the chiasm of animals with forward-facing eyes: here axons from the nasal half of the retina decussate, but the temporal fibres remain ipsilateral, presumably to allow images of an object seen in both eyes to be processed together in higher visual areas. Recent work suggests that whatever guidance mechanisms are responsible for partial decussation at the chiasm, they may be imperfect, because initially many axons take mistaken routes towards the inappropriate side of the brain (Land & Lund, 1979) or even towards the other eye (Bunt & Lund, 1981). Some of these aberrant axons are removed by cell death (see chapter IV.1). Curiously decussation of the optic nerves in adult albino animals is more complete than in normal adults, and the pigmented cells which albinos lack appear to be important in

Fig. III.3. Left: projections of normal eye and ventral–ventral compound eye to the optic tecta of *Xenopus*. Axons from the compound eye select a restricted pathway to the tectum. C, caudal; L, lateral; M, medial; R, rostral; d, dorsal; n, nasal; t, temporal; v, ventral. Right: surface view of *Xenopus* brain to show position of tectum.

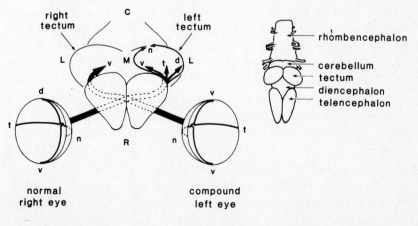

guiding the retinal axons in the optic nerve (Silver & Sapiro, 1981). However, there are no gross differences between albino and normal rats in the initial retino-collicular projections (Land & Lund, 1979), so the role of pigmented cells in guidance is still unclear.

Innervation of sympathetic ganglia

In 1897 Langley reported that a cut preganglionic nerve regenerated into the superior cervical ganglion and that normal function was restored to the sympathetic end-organs. He suggested that a selective reinnervation of ganglion cells had occurred, brought about by a chemical matching of pre- and post-ganglionic neurons with the same function. Recent study of this phenomenon of target recognition has shown that ganglion cells are innervated and reinnervated preferentially by preganglionic axons that arise from three or four contiguous segmental levels of the cord (Nja & Purves, 1977*a*, *b*). Segmental specificity is also displayed in the reinnervation of thoracic and lumbar ganglia transplanted in place of the superior cervical ganglion: cells in the transplanted ganglia are innervated more effectively by axons in the preganglionic trunk arising from more caudal spinal nerves (Purves, Thompson & Yip, 1981). A similar specificity is exhibited when the preganglionic nerve is made to innervate *intercostal muscles* from different thoracic levels (Wigston & Sanes, 1982).

These interesting observations hint of graded segmental labels exhibited in common by a variety of tissues. In the superior cervical ganglion in particular, it appears that different cells carry different segmental labels, probably in addition to function-specific labels. It is possible that the labels are imprinted on the ganglion cells by the preganglionic terminals, just as labels may be imprinted on the tectum. Alternatively the labels might be induced retrogradely on the cell bodies when the axons of the cells first contact the various target organs. This would be a logical extension of the hypothesis that transmitter phenotypes of crest cells are specified by local environmental influences (see chapter II.1). If it is so, then the induced labels must become permanent in the adult, because they are not respecified when the post-ganglionic axons regenerate to different target organs (Purves & Thompson, 1979). One other possibility is that the labels exist on the ganglion cells before pre- and post-synaptic innervation occurs. The labels would then be responsible for establishing the specificity of presynaptic connections by a mechanism of target recognition. Such labels would be unlikely to be conferred by spatial gradients in the ganglion, because ganglion cells that innervate particular target organs are scattered throughout the ganglion (Lichtman, Purves & Yip, 1979). The labels would therefore have to be specified probably before the cells migrate to the ganglion.

Pioneer fibres and 'stepping stones' in insects

In insects the first axons to grow along the future branches of the peripheral nerves are produced by a few identifiable sensory neurons in the limb buds. These pioneer fibres grow into the CNS and are joined subsequently by other sensory axons arising from nearby neurons. Axons from the CNS also grow out into the periphery along the developing nerve bundles.

As they grow towards the CNS the pioneer fibres make characteristic sharp changes of direction, a behaviour that is not compatible with the smoothly directed growth that might be expected along chemotactic gradients (fig. III.4). Bate (1976) proposed that the sharp turns were made at the sites of specific target cells or 'stepping stones'. The stepping stones have been identified recently as cells which bind antibodies specific to neurons, and these cells subsequently produce axons which join the peripheral nerves. The filopodia of the pioneer growth cones can be longer than the distance between these cells, and the filopodia do not appear to be guided in their initial extensions. It is therefore likely that the guidance of pioneers occurs by undirected filopodial exploration followed by contact with, recognition of, and growth towards the stepping stone or 'guidepost' neurons (see review by Bentley & Keshishian, 1982). This could be regarded as guidance by sequential target recognition.

Destruction of some pioneer neurons with a laser beam can disrupt the normal pattern of peripheral nerve development (Edwards, Chen & Berns, 1981), but it is also clear that other neurons can navigate the pioneer pathway in the absence of the normal pioneers (Bentley & Keshishian,

Fig. III.4. Establishment of pathways to CNS by pioneer fibres in insect leg.

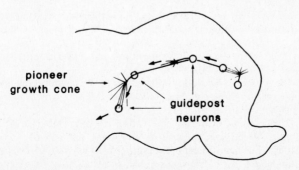

1982). The pioneer neurons thus probably do not have a unique pathfinding ability, but are simply the first to produce axons and to come into contact with the nearby guidepost neurons. The affinity between pioneers and guideposts probably exists between all the neurons and their axons in the limb and is likely to be responsible for axons 'fasciculating' together into bundles.

References

Guidance pathways

Katz, M.J. & Lasek, R.J. (1978). Eyes transplanted to tadpole tails send axons rostrally in two spinal cord tracts. *Science*, **199**, 202–3.

Katz, M.J., Lasek, R.J. & Nauta, H.J.W. (1980). Ontogeny of substrate pathways and the origin of the neural circuit pattern. *Neuroscience*, **5**, 821–33.

Menesini-Chen, M.G., Chen, J.S. & Levi-Montalcini, R. (1978). Sympathetic nerve fibres ingrowth in the CNS of neonatal rodent upon intracerebral NGF injections. *Archives italiennes de biologie*, **116**, 53–84.

Silver, J., Lorenz, S.E., Wahlsten, D. & Coughlin, J. (1982). Axonal guidance during development of the great cerebral commissures: descriptive and experimental studies, *in vivo*, on the role of preformed pathways. *Journal of Comparative Neurology*, **210**, 10–29.

Singer, M., Norlander, R.H. & Egar, M. (1979). Axonal guidance during embryogenesis and regeneration in the spinal cord of the newt: the blueprint hypothesis of neuronal pathway patterning. *Journal of Comparative Neurology*, **185**, 1–22.

Summerbell, D. & Stirling, R.V. (1981). The innervation of dorso-ventrally reversed chick wings: evidence that motor axons do not actively seek out their appropriate targets. *Journal of Embryology and Experimental Morphology*, **61**, 233–47.

Innervation of limbs

Dennis, M.J. & Yip, J.W. (1978). Formation and elimination of foreign synapses on adult salamander muscle. *Journal of Physiology*, **274**, 299–310.

Frank, E., Jansen, J.K.S., Lømo, T. & Westgaard, R.H. (1975). The interaction between foreign and original motor nerves innervating the soleus muscle of rats. *Journal of Physiology*, **247**, 725–43.

Gerding, R., Robbins, N. & Antosiak, J. (1977). Efficiency of reinnervation of neonatal rat muscle by original and foreign nerves. *Developmental Biology*, **61**, 177–83.

Grimm, C.M. (1971). An evaluation of myotypic respecification in axolotls. *Journal of Experimental Zoology*, **178**, 479–96.

Heidemann, M.K. (1977). Neurophysiological and behavioural evidence for selective reinnervation of skin-grafted *Rana pipiens*. *Proceedings of the National Academy of Sciences, USA*, **74**, 5749–53.

Hollyday, M. (1981). Rules of motor innervation in chick embryos with supernumerary limbs. *Journal of Comparative Neurology*, **202**, 439–65.

Honig, M.G. (1982). The development of sensory projection patterns in embryonic chick hind limbs. *Journal of Physiology*, **330**, 175–202.

Lamb, A.H. (1977). Neuronal death in the development of the somatotopic projections of the ventral horn in *Xenopus*. *Brain Research*, **134**, 145–50.

Lance-Jones, C. & Landmesser, L. (1980). Motoneurone projection patterns in the chick hind limb following early partial reversals of the spinal cord. *Journal of Physiology*, **302**, 581–602.

Lance-Jones, C. & Landmesser, L. (1981). Pathway selection by chick lumbosacal motoneurons in an experimentally altered environment. *Proceedings of the Royal Society of London, Series B*, **214**, 19–52.

Landmesser, L. (1978). The development of motor projection patterns in the chick hind limb. *Journal of Physiology*, **284**, 391–414.

Landmesser, L. & Honig, M.G. (1982). The effect of motoneuron removal on sensory neuron outgrowth in chick hindlimb. *Society of Neuroscience Abstracts*, **8**, 929.

Lewis, J., Chevallier, A., Kieny, M. & Wolpert, L. (1981). Muscle nerves do not develop in chick wings devoid of muscle. *Journal of Embryology and Experimental Morphology*, **64**, 211–32.

Miner, N. (1956). Integumental specification of sensory fibres in the development of cutaneous local sign. *Journal of Comparative Neurology*, **105**, 161–71.

Scott, S.A. (1982). The development of the segmental pattern of skin sensory innervation in embryonic chick hind limb. *Journal of Physiology*, **330**, 203–20.

Summerbell, D. & Stirling, R.V. (1981). The innervation of dorso-ventrally reversed chick wings: evidence that motor axons do not actively seek out their appropriate targets. *Journal of Embryology and Experimental Morphology*, **61**, 233–47.

Projection of retina to tectum

Barbera, A.J., Marchase, R.B. & Roth, S. (1973). Adhesive recognition and retinotectal specificity. *Proceedings of the National Academy of Sciences, USA*, **70**, 2482–6.

Bunt, S.M. & Lund, R.D. (1981). Development of a transient retino-retinal pathway in hooded and albino rats. *Brain Research*, **211**, 399–404.

Chung, S.M. & Cooke, J. (1978). Observations on the formation of the brain and of nerve connections following embryonic manipulation of the amphibian neural tube. *Proceedings of the Royal Society of London, Series B*, **201**, 335–73.

Fawcett, J.W. (1981). How axons grow down the *Xenopus* optic nerve. *Journal of Embryology and Experimental Morphology*, **65**, 219–33.

Fujisawa, H. (1981). Retinotopic analysis of fibre pathways in the regenerating retinotectal system of the adult newt, *Cynops pyrrhyogaster*. *Brain Research*, **206**, 27–37.

Gaze, R.M. (1974). Neuronal specificity. *British Medical Bulletin*, **30**, 116–21.

Gaze, R.M., Keating, M.J., Ostberg, A. & Chung, S.-H. (1979). The relationship between retinal and tectal growth in larval *Xenopus*: implications for the development of the retinotectal projection. *Journal of Embryology and Experimental Morphology*, **53**, 103–43.

Hope, R.A., Hammond, B.J. & Gaze, R.M. (1976). The arrow model: retinotectal specificity and map formation in the goldfish visual system. *Proceedings of the Royal Society of London, Series B*, **194**, 447–66.

Land, P.W. & Lund, R.D. (1979). Development of the rat's uncrossed retinotectal pathway and its relation to plasticity studies. *Science*, **205**, 698–700.

Meyer, R.L. (1980). Mapping the normal and regenerating retinotectal projection of goldfish with autoradiographic methods. *Journal of Comparative Neurology*, **189**, 273–89.

Schmidt, J.T. (1978). Retinal fibres alter tectal positional markers during the expansion of the half retinal projection in goldfish. *Journal of Comparative Neurology*, **177**, 279–300.

Schmidt, J.T. (1982). The formation of retinotectal projections. *Trends in Neurosciences*, **5**, 111–15.

Scholes, J.H. (1979). Nerve fibre topography in the retinal projection to the tectum. *Nature, London*, **278**, 620–4.

Silver, J. & Sapiro, J. (1981). Axonal guidance during development of the optic nerve: the role of pigmented epithelia and other extrinsic factors. *Journal of Comparative Neurology*, **202**, 521–38.

Sperry, R.W. (1943). Effects of 180 degree rotation of the retinal field on visuo-motor co-ordination. *Journal of Experimental Zoology*, **92**, 263–79.

Straznicky, C., Gaze, R.M. & Keating, M.J. (1981). The development of the retinotectal projections from compound eyes in *Xenopus*. *Journal of Embryology and Experimental Morphology*, **62**, 13–35.

Trisler, G.D., Schneider, M.D. & Nirenberg, M. (1981). A topographic gradient of molecules in retina can be used to identify neuron position. *Proceedings of the National Academy of Sciences, USA*, **78**, 2145–9.

Innervation of sympathetic ganglia

Langley, J.N. (1897). On the regeneration of pre-ganglionic and post-ganglionic visceral nerve fibres. *Journal of Physiology*, **22**, 215–30.

Lichtman, J.W., Purves, D. & Yip, J.W. (1979). On the purpose of selective innervation of guinea-pig superior cervical ganglion cells. *Journal of Physiology*, **292**, 69–84.

Nja, A. & Purves, D. (1977*a*). Specific innervation of guinea-pig superior cervical ganglion cells by pre-ganglionic fibres arising from different levels of the spinal cord. *Journal of Physiology*, **264**, 565–83.

Nja, A. & Purves, D. (1977*b*). Reinnervation of guinea-pig superior cervical ganglion cells by pre-ganglionic fibres arising from different levels of the spinal cord. *Journal of Physiology*, **272**, 633–51.

Purves, D. & Thompson, W. (1979). The effects of post-ganglionic axotomy on selective sympathetic connections in the superior cervical ganglion of the guinea-pig. *Journal of Physiology*, **297**, 95–110.

Purves, D., Thompson, W. & Yip, J.W. (1981). Reinnervation of ganglia transplanted to the neck from different levels of the guinea-pig sympathetic chain. *Journal of Physiology*, **313**, 49–63.

Wigston, D.J. & Sanes, J.R. (1982). Selective reinnervation of adult mammalian muscle by axons from different segmental levels. *Nature, London*, **299**, 464–7.

Pioneer fibres and 'stepping stones' in insects

Bate, C.M. (1976). Pioneer neurons in the insect embryo. *Nature, London*, **260**, 54–6.

Bentley, D. & Keshishian, H. (1982). Pioneer neurons and pathways in insect appendages. *Trends in Neurosciences*, **5**, 354–8.

Edwards, J.S., Chen, S.-W. & Berns, M.W. (1981). Cercal sensory development following laser microlesions of embryonic apical cells in *Achita domesticus*. *Journal of Neuroscience*, **1**, 250–8.

III.3

Development of axon–target and axon–glia cell contacts

Synaptogenesis

Synapse formation requires the incoming axon to change from a state of growth to that appropriate for release of transmitter from a stationary terminal. In the post-synaptic cell, changes appropriate for receiving transmitter occur in the region of membrane apposed to the nerve terminal, and extrajunctional membrane properties are also modified, probably to localise synaptic growth. These changes are accompanied by the development of structural specialisations in the pre- and post-synaptic cells.

Although some observations on the development of synapses in ganglia and the CNS have been made, these are for the most part only descriptive; synaptogenesis at the neuromuscular junction has been subjected to much more experimentation in attempts to identify and characterise each step in the process. The major contributions have come from three sorts of experiment: regeneration of synapses in adults when a nerve grows back to its original synaptic sites; synapse formation at new sites on denervated adult muscle fibres; and formation of synapses between embryonic nerve and muscle cells in tissue culture.

Presynaptic differentiation

When adult muscles are reinnervated following nerve crush it is more usual for axons to terminate again at old synaptic sites rather than to form new 'ectopic' synapses. Sanes, Marshall & McMahan (1978) showed that in the frog the recognition marker which acts as a 'stop signal' is in the basal lamina overlying the junction, because it is effective even when the muscle cell underlying it has degenerated. This suggests that there may be areas on the surface of target cells which act as recognition sites by inhibiting growth cone activity in the arriving axons. It is known that clusters of acetylcholine receptors occur in embryonic or denervated muscle membrane, but it is not clear whether axons stop at these clusters (Frank & Fischbach, 1979), or stop at sites they have induced themselves (see below), or stop at other specialised sites which may be present in the central region of the muscle before axons arrive (Harris, 1981). The subcellular basis for the inhibition of growth is not known. The most likely mechanisms include: active inhibition of growth mediated by contact with the junctional basal lamina; a change in the property of the extrajunctional basal lamina which makes it unsuitable for nerve growth; and decreased release by the muscle of a diffusible growth stimulus.

Transmitter can be released from an axon terminal as it first comes into contact with its post-synaptic cell (e.g. De Cino, 1981). As the terminal matures transmitter is released by exocytosis at specialised active zones which in the neuromuscular junction are in register with the clefts between the tops of the secondary folds of the post-synaptic membrane. The signal for formation of the release sites is also found in the basal lamina, since the release sites re-form when nerves regenerate into a muscle in which only the basal laminal sheaths remain (Sanes *et al.*, 1978). Full development of the presynaptic release mechanism requires matching not only of transmitter–receptor partners, but also of positionally compatible pre- and post-synaptic cells: in frogs, for example, less transmitter is released by the terminals of motor neurons when they reinnervate a wrong muscle rather than their own muscle (Sayers & Tonge, 1982). Transmitter release and other aspects of the development of the presynaptic terminal may also be influenced by growth factors released by the target and taken up by the nerve terminal: for example NGF uptake by sympathetic ganglion cells can change transmitter output by increasing production of transmitter-synthesising enzymes (Thoenen *et al.*, 1971). As yet, evidence that similar substances might act on other nerve cell terminals is indirect (see part IV).

Post-synaptic differentiation

There is now strong evidence that the accumulation of transmitter receptors at the neuromuscular junction, which initially involves lateral migration of receptors from surrounding muscle areas (Anderson & Cohen, 1977), is caused by a substance liberated from or attached to nerve terminals. First, if both nerve and muscle cells are killed, a chemical marker which is left behind in the junctional basal lamina can induce receptor accumulation in myotubes regenerating within the intact lamina (Burden,

Sargent & McMahan, 1979). Secondly, even degenerating nerves which have made only brief contact with muscle before axotomy leave behind a marker which stimulates receptor accumulation at extrajunctional sites on denervated muscle (Lømo & Slater, 1980). Thirdly, a factor has been isolated from neural tissues which increases receptor aggregation on cultured muscle cells (e.g. Bauer *et al.*, 1981). The factor responsible is not exhibited on all nerve cells, because neither sensory nor sympathetic nerves will induce aggregation of acetylcholine receptors on muscle cells in culture (Cohen & Weldon, 1980). It is implicit in these findings that receptor accumulation occurs in the absence of electrical activity, and this has been confirmed for synapse development *in vivo* and *in vitro* (e.g. Cohen, 1972).

Components of the post-synaptic membrane can be detected in muscle cells in culture in the complete absence of nerve. The most obvious of these components is of course the acetylcholine receptor, but the junctional form of cholinesterase is also present on myotubes of a muscle cell line, and antisera raised against synapses bind specifically to these muscle cells (Silberstein, Inestrosa & Hall, 1982). It is likely, then, that the presynaptic nerve does not instruct the muscle to begin synthesis of new junctional components, but instead regulates the synthesis and siting of existing components.

The subsequent events in neuromuscular synaptogenesis include, in the approximate order of their occurrence: accumulation of acetylcholinesterase in the basal lamina at the junction; loss of the ability of non-innervated membrane to accept innervation; stabilisation (increase in half-life) of receptors in the clusters; decrease in the open time of the transmitter-activated ion channels; elimination of transmitter receptors from extra-junctional membrane; and development of synaptic folds. In rats and chicks cholinesterase activity begins to develop at sites of nerve contact only when the muscle is activated (see e.g. Lømo & Slater, 1980) but in toads activity may not be required (Weldon, Moody-Corbett & Cohen, 1981). Activity of the muscle has been shown to be the key factor in suppressing the formation of receptors elsewhere in the muscle (Lømo & Rosenthal, 1972) and making the muscle refractory to further innervation (Jansen *et al.*, 1973). Receptor stabilisation occurs before birth in rats whereas ion channel properties change in the following weeks, possibly as existing receptors pack more densely (Michler & Sakmann, 1980). Finally, actin is present at junctions (Hall, Lubit & Schwartz, 1981) and may be involved in production and stabilisation of the synaptic folds, which develop only if a muscle is active (T.P. Feng, unpublished).

Much less is known about events in the development of synapses elsewhere in the nervous system, which may differ from the neuromuscular junction in important aspects. For example, post-synaptic structures can develop in the absence of their presynaptic axons in ganglia (Smolen, 1981) and in the cerebellum (see chapter III.1).

A summary of the findings on the development of the neuromuscular junction is given in fig. III.5. Acetylcholine receptors accumulate at a site which is most probably induced by contact with the nerve. This site is the nerve's 'toehold' on the surface, which elsewhere become inhospitable with the onset of electrical activity. Activity plays a necessary part in many of the steps in synaptogenesis subsequent to the accumulation of receptors. The effects of activity are presumably brought about by as yet unidentified changes in metabolism of the muscle cell. It is not known whether transmitter or other substances released by the nerve have additional direct effects on post-synaptic development.

Sensory receptor formation

The peripheral terminals of most sensory axons are closely associated with specialised receptor cells that take part in transducing a sensory stimulus into electrical impulses. The presence of the sensory nerve is essential for the normal development of the sensory end-organs. Muscle spindles, for example, cannot be detected in the adult rat if the afferents are removed at birth (Zelena, 1964). In the case of innervation of Merkel cells

Fig. III.5. Development of the neuromuscular junction. Events marked with an asterisk (*) require post-synaptic activity. ACh, acetylcholine.

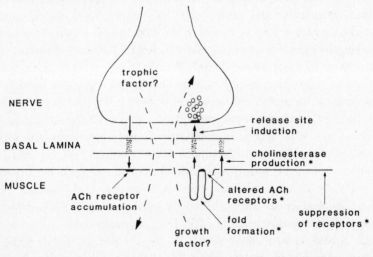

(specialised touch receptors in the skin) it is known that the receptor cells exist before arrival of the nerve and can develop partially in the nerve's absence (Scott, Cooper & Diamond, 1981). The Merkel cell afferent seeks out its target either by chemotropism or by random searching and recognition (English, Burgess & Norman, 1980).

Other sensory targets may also exist before sensory nerves arrive, or there may be induction of specialised receptor cells from uncommitted cells in the target area. It is possible, for example, that myotubes contacted by spindle sensory axons are induced to develop into the specialised muscle fibres of the spindle, while myotubes contacted by motor axons develop into normal muscle fibres. The spindle's motor axons probably seek out the developing spindle, since they apparently make their first contact with the spindle at least several days behind the sensory axons (Milburn, 1973). Definitive experiments to determine the nature of the signal from sensory nerves that causes either induction or subsequent differentiation of the receptor cells are still lacking. (See also the sections on trophic effects, chapter IV.4.)

Neuron–glia relationships

Glial cells proliferate as they migrate out into the periphery along the developing peripheral nerves. The additional glial cells are probably generated to maintain adequate numbers to ensheath the axons. Cultures of purified nerve cells and purified glial cells isolated from embryonic ganglia have been used to show that glial cell division is stimulated only by contact with the nerve cell membrane (Salzer, Bunge & Glaser, 1980). Cultures of glial cells have also been used to identify a mitogenic factor in adult brain which exists in relatively high concentration in the pituitary; its significance for development is not yet clear (Brockes, Lemke & Balzer, 1980).

The differentiation of glial cells following their proliferation is probably also controlled by axons. In peripheral nerves the larger axons become myelinated by their glial cells while the smaller axons remain unmyelinated. If myelinated nerves are cross-sutured with the distal segment of an unmyelinated nerve, the regenerating axons will become myelinated, whereas an unmyelinated nerve regenerating into a previously myelinated nerve remains unmyelinated (Simpson & Young, 1945). This means that the axons, rather than the glial cells, control the myelination. The signal for myelination may be in part causally related to axon diameter, since there is a good correlation between degree of myelination and diameter (Friede, 1972). The differentiation of CNS glial cells can occur *in vitro*, and it is stimulated by a protein extracted from brain (Lim *et al.*, 1977). It is not yet known whether this protein is made by nerve cells or whether it is involved in glial differentiation in the CNS.

Schwann cells in their turn appear to influence the differentiation of axons during development. The excitable membrane of the axon is restricted to the nodal region of myelinated nerves by the Schwann cells, because saltatory conduction does not develop in axons if glial cells are absent, and is replaced by continuous conduction if mature axons are demyelinated with diphtheria toxin (Bostock & Sears, 1978). (For a full review of axon–glia relationships in development see Bray, Rasminsky & Aguayo, 1981.)

Conclusion to part III

Spaces in tissues, gradients of diffusible substances, and gradients or discrete differences in the properties of cell surfaces seem to be the main factors guiding the growth cones of axons and dendrites through surrounding tissues. Axon growth cones are guided to the immediate vicinity of their target cells, where there is a contact-mediated recognition interaction that permits synapses to form only between appropriately matched partners. Subsequent development of synapses occurs as a result of chemical and electrical interactions between axon and target cell.

The guidance and recognition mechanisms do not appear to be completely accurate, because the initial patterns of connections are subsequently modified. The ways in which these and other modifications are achieved are considered in part IV.

References

Synaptogenesis

Anderson, M.J. & Cohen, M.W. (1977). Nerve-induced and spontaneous redistribution of acetylcholine receptors on cultured muscle cells. *Journal of Physiology*, **268**, 757–73.

Bauer, H.C., Daniels, M.P., Pudimat, P.A., Jacques, L., Sugiyama, H. & Christian, C.N. (1981). Characterisation and partial purification of a neuronal factor which increases acetylcholine receptor aggregation on cultured muscle cells. *Brain Research*, **209**, 395–404.

Burden, S.J., Sargent, P.B. & McMahan, U.J. (1979). Acetylcholine receptors in regenerating muscle accumulate at original synaptic sites in the absence of the nerve. *Journal of Cell Biology*, **82**, 412–25.

Cohen, M.W. (1972). The development of neurotransmitter connections in the presence of D-tubocurarine. *Brain Research*, **41**, 457–63.

Cohen, M.W. & Weldon, P.R. (1980). Localization of acetylcholine receptors and synaptic ultrastructure at nerve–muscle contacts in culture: dependence on nerve type. *Journal of Cell Biology*, **86**, 388–401.

De Cino, P. (1981). Transmitter release properties along regenerated nerve processes. *Journal of Neuroscience*, **1**, 308–17.

Frank, E. & Fischbach, G.D. (1979). Early events in neuromuscular junction formation *in vitro*. *Journal of Cell Biology*, **83**, 145–58.

Hall, Z.W., Lubit, B.W. & Schwartz, J.H. (1981). Cytoplasmic actin in postsynaptic structures at the neuromuscular junction. *Journal of Cell Biology*, **90**, 789–92.

Harris, A.J. (1981). Embryonic growth and innervation of rat skeletal muscles. III. Neural regulation of junctional and extrajunctional acetylcholine receptor clusters. *Philosophical Transactions of the Royal Society of London, Series B*, **293**, 287–314.

Jansen, J.K.S., Lømo, T., Nicolaysen, T. & Westgaard, R.H. (1973). Hyperinnervation of skeletal muscle fibres: dependence on muscle activity. *Science*, **181**, 559–61.

Lømo, T. & Rosenthal, J. (1972). Control of acetylcholine sensitivity by muscle activity in the rat. *Journal of Physiology*, **221**, 493–513.

Lømo, T. & Slater, C.R. (1980). Control of junctional acetylcholinesterase by neural and muscular influences in the rat. *Journal of Physiology*, **303**, 191–202.

Michler, A. & Sakmann, B. (1980). Receptor stability and channel conversion in the subsynaptic membrane of the developing mammalian neuromuscular junction. *Developmental Biology*, **80**, 1–17.

Sanes, J.R., Marshall, L.M. & McMahan, U.J. (1978). Reinnervation of muscle fibre basal lamina after removal of myofibres. *Journal of Cell Biology*, **78**, 176–98.

Sayers, H. & Tonge, D.A. (1982). Differences between foreign and original innervation of skeletal muscle in the frog. *Journal of Physiology*, **330**, 57–68.

Silberstein, L., Inestrosa, N.C. & Hall, Z.W. (1982). Aneural muscle cell cultures make synaptic basal lamina components. *Nature, London*, **295**, 143–5.

Smolen, A.J. (1981). Postnatal development of ganglionic neurons in the absence of preganglionic input: morphological observations on synaptic formation. *Developmental Brain Research*, **1**, 49–58.

Thoenen, H., Angeletti, P.V., Levi-Montalcini, R. & Kettler, R. (1971). Selective-induction by nerve growth factor of tyrosine hydroxylase and dopamine-β-hydroxylase in the rat superior cervical ganglia. *Proceedings of the National Academy of Sciences, USA*, **68**, 1598–602.

Weldon, P.R., Moody-Corbett, F. & Cohen, M.W. (1981). Ultrastructure of sites of cholinesterase activity on amphibian embryonic muscle cells cultured without nerve. *Developmental Biology*, **84**, 341–50.

Sensory receptor formation

English, K.B., Burgess, P.R. & Norman, D.K. v. (1980). Development of rat Merkel cells. *Journal of Comparative Neurology*, **194**, 475–96.

Milburn, A. (1973). The early development of muscle spindles in the rat. *Journal of Cell Science*, **12**, 175–95.

Scott, S.A., Cooper, E. & Diamond, J. (1981). Merkel cells as targets of the mechanosensory nerves in salamander skin. *Proceedings of the Royal Society of London, Series B,* **211**, 455–70.

Zelena, J. (1964). Development, degeneration and regeneration of receptor organs. *Progress in Brain Research,* **13**, 175–213.

Neuron–glia relationships

Bostock, H. & Sears, T.A. (1978). The internodal axon membrane: electrical excitability and continuous conduction in segmental demyelination. *Journal of Physiology,* **280**, 273–301.

Bray, G.M., Rasminsky, M. & Aguayo, A.J. (1981). Interaction between axons and their sheath cells. *Annual Review of Neuroscience,* **4**, 127–62.

Brockes, J., Lemke, G.E. & Balzer, D.R. (1980). Purification and preliminary characterisation of a glial growth factor from the bovine pituitary. *Journal of Biological Chemistry,* **255**, 8374–7.

Friede, R.L. (1972). Control of myelin formation by axon caliber (with a model of the control mechanism). *Journal of Comparative Neurology,* **144**, 233–52.

Lim, R., Turriff, D.E., Troy, S.S., Moore, B.W. & Eng, L.F. (1977). Glial maturation factor: effect on chemical differentiation of glioblasts in culture. *Science,* **195**, 195–6.

Salzer, J.L., Bunge, R.P. & Glaser, L. (1980). Studies of Schwann cell proliferation. III. Evidence for the surface localisation of the neurite mitogen. *Journal of Cellular Biology,* **84**, 767–78.

Simpson, S.A. & Young, J.Z. (1945). Regeneration of fibre diameter after cross unions of visceral and somatic nerves. *Journal of Anatomy,* **79**, 48–65.

PART IV
Modification of connections

Synopsis

As synapses begin to form, considerable modifications occur in the pattern of connections between nerve and target cells. The first of these modifications is neuronal death, which removes a variable but usually large proportion of the neurons which have sent out axons to their targets. Cell death probably eliminates errors in the initial pattern of connections and matches pre- and post-synaptic cell numbers. The mechanism underlying neuronal cell death is not fully understood, but it may depend upon electrical activity in the nerve–target pathways and involve uptake by the neurons of substances essential for their survival. One of the substances required for the survival of sympathetic neurons and dorsal root ganglion cells is the well-known Nerve Growth Factor.

When axons reach their targets they branch extensively and contact more post-synaptic cells than they do in the adult. Some axons also produce superfluous collateral branches that make unused contacts with other targets. The elimination of these excess connections after the period of cell death is the second major phase in the modification of connections. Excess connections have been found in muscles, ganglia and at various loci in the CNS. The mechanism for their elimination, like that for cell death, is dependent upon electrical activity, and competition between the axon terminals for a factor may also be involved.

During this stage of development it has been found that many neuronal connections are easily and permanently modified by alterations in the normal patterns of neural activity induced by environmental stimuli. This phenomenon has been studied extensively in the mammalian visual cortex, where it is found that abnormal visual experience produces abnormally responding neurons. The changes in the response properties of the neurons can be brought about most readily during a certain relatively short time interval, the so-called critical period. The neuroanatomical basis for critical periods is probably the presence of the excess and widespread presynaptic nerve branches, which provide an initial diffuse array of connections out of which the normal adult pattern can be sculpted. It is likely that presynaptic inputs which release transmitter in close synchrony with firing of post-synaptic cells are the ones which survive.

After the critical period neuronal connections, whether normal or abnormal, become much more permanent. However, in the adult some neuronal pathways must change in response to experience in order to account for the phenomena of learning and memory. This modifiability of the adult brain is referred to as plasticity. Several convenient pathways in the adult mammalian CNS have been found where plasticity can be readily demonstrated and studied, notably pathways in the hippocampus, red nucleus and cerebellum, and pathways mediating the vestibulo-ocular reflex. The synaptic modifications in pathways mediating a modifiable reflex response in a sea snail have also been studied with great success. The basis of adult plasticity appears to be the modification of converging inputs that are synchronously active.

Interactions between nerves and their target and glial cells continue to occur following the establishment of the relatively stable pattern of connections in the adult. The axon is the link between the nerve cell and the other cells involved, and transection of the axon interrupts the interactions and causes regressive changes in nerve, target and glial cells. These interactions have been described as *trophic* influences (from the Greek *trophe*, meaning food or sustenance) because they are necessary for maintaining the cell properties associated with the innervated state. Trophic interactions occur in both the orthograde direction (the nerve maintaining its target and glial cells) and the retrograde direction (the target and glial cells maintaining the nerve). Trophic interactions in the adult are important in relation to development of the nervous system in that they probably represent the continued operation of mechanisms which bring about the development of innervation.

The final chapter in this part of the book deals with changes in connections that occur following injury to the nervous system. These changes usually involve regrowth of damaged axons and sprouting of remaining intact axons and terminals in the vicinity of the degenerating nerves, and both forms of growth can reinnervate and restore function to denervated cells. The development of the new outgrowths appears to be controlled partly by the reversion of the denervated tissues to an embryonic state which can stimulate nerve growth and accept innervation, and also by the availability of suitable pathways for the sprouting or regenerating nerves to follow. Changes in the nerve cell body appropriate for producing new growth may also occur. In addition to activation of new growth, injury can activate synapses which under normal circumstances are physiologically suppressed or undetectable.

IV.1

Nerve cell death

Most of the different types of neuron in the vertebrate nervous system are subject to a period of cell death, which occurs shortly after axons begin to reach and activate their targets (Hamburger & Oppenheim, 1982). The extent of cell death for a given type of neuron is determined from estimates of the absolute number of neurons at a given site at different developmental stages. The number of neurons is found first to rise to a maximum as neurons proliferate and settle at their final destination, then to decline with the onset of cell death, and finally to reach a plateau when the period of death has passed. Death of the neurons is confirmed by the presence of degenerating nerve cell bodies during the decline in numbers of normal cells.

The proportion of cells that die varies in the different parts of the nervous system. Death eliminates only a small fraction of the neurons at some sites but extensive death eliminating at least half of the total number of neurons generated is more usual. Cell death is thus a major event in neuronal development, and there has been a succession of hypotheses about the purpose it might serve. The evidence discussed below points to cell death acting to leave behind only those neurons with enough suitable pre- and post-synaptic connections. This seemingly wasteful process appears to have evolved in preference to accurate generation of neuron numbers and precise guidance of outgrowing axons (see Clarke, 1981).

Specific proteins derived from target tissues are necessary for the survival of different kinds of embryonic neuron in tissue culture, and there is now convincing evidence that one of these proteins, Nerve Growth Factor, is required for the survival of sympathetic and sensory neurons in the animal. Activity in the nerve–target pathways is another important part of the mechanism underlying cell death, and this may modulate the production and uptake of the survival factors.

Neuronal death also occurs in invertebrates, apparently to remove neurons that lack a target or that receive inadequate presynaptic connections. However, the mechanism underlying invertebrate neuronal death is not yet clear.

Purpose of cell death

Nerve cell death was first observed in sensory ganglia and in motor neurons in the ventral horn of the spinal cord of chick embryos following removal of limb buds before they become innervated. This produced a virtually complete degeneration of all the nerve cells which had been deprived of their targets in the limb (see Hamburger, 1980, for a review). When cell death in normal embryos was subsequently discovered in ganglia and the spinal cord (Hamburger & Levi-Montalcini, 1949), it was found to occur at the same time as the induced cell death and differed only in being less extensive. This suggested that the neurons that die are simply those that fail to reach a suitable target. This attractively simple idea may well account for neuronal death at some sites in the nervous system. For example, the sympathetic preganglionic motor neurons are generated as a uniform column of cells (the columns of Terni) on each side of the spinal cord, but at the cervical level they appear to lack a target and subsequently degenerate. If the cervical cord is transplanted to the thoracic level some of the cells succeed in innervating ganglia and survive (Shieh, 1951). However, it has also been found that horseradish peroxidase (HRP) injected into target tissues of somatic motor neurons and parasympathetic neurons just before cell death occurs can be detected subsequently in cells that die (Lamb, 1976; Landmesser & Pilar, 1976). This means that failure to reach a suitable target cannot be the only reason for cell death.

Neuronal death in the sensory ganglia and cord at segmental levels which innervate the limbs is less extensive than at the levels which innervate the trunk regions, where there is much less tissue to be innervated. Moreover if extra limbs are grafted onto early embryos there is less neuronal death at the levels innervating the extra limb (Hollyday & Hamburger, 1976). These observations are consistent with the hypothesis that a given target tissue in some way supports the survival of only a limited number of the neurons that initially innervate it. Thus, cell death could be a means of matching appropriately the sizes of independently generated pre- and post-synaptic cell populations by limiting survival of the presynaptic cells (Cowan, 1973).

Death could similarly eliminate post-synaptic cells if these were generated in relative excess over the numbers of presynaptic neurons (fig. IV.1).

Observations on the death of retinal ganglion cells in neonatal rats following injury to the optic nerve suggest that both post-synaptic and presynaptic population matching may regulate the survival of these cells (fig. IV.2). Severing the optic nerve before the chiasm, reduces death in the other eye in the ganglion cells which project ipsilaterally from the temporal retina, presumably because removal of the axon terminals of one eye leaves relatively more target for the remaining axons (Jeffery & Perry, 1982). Section of the optic tract on the central side of the chiasm also leads to less death in the same ganglion cells, in this case possibly because these cells receive more presynaptic input from the other neurons in the retina following the degeneration of the injured neurons (Linden & Perry, 1982).

A test of whether motor neuron death is responsible for matching the size of motor neuron pools to their presynaptic inputs has recently been carried out by Oppenheim and his coworkers, who eliminated sensory inputs by excising the neural crest and also removed other descending inputs by transecting the spinal cord (Okada & Oppenheim, 1981). In both cases the usual phase of cell death was unaffected, which implies that presynaptic inputs do not influence survival of motor neurons. An experiment by Lamb (1980) has also cast doubt on the idea that death reduces motor neuron

Fig. IV.1. Possible matching of pre- and post-synaptic cell populations by cell death (1:1 matching shown here for simplicity).

excess presynaptic cells

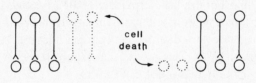

excess post-synaptic cells

Fig. IV.2. Reduced cell death in temporal retina following neonatal transection of either optic nerve (left) or optic tract (right).

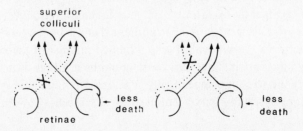

pool sizes to match the size of their targets. Lamb succeeded in diverting the outgrowing nerves from one side of the spinal cord into the developing contralateral leg in tadpoles. The result was a normal-sized leg musculature innervated by twice as many motor neurons, but surprisingly there was no increase in the amount of cell death on either side of the cord. This result needs to be confirmed in other species and with variations in target size (e.g. by the use of limb-switched avian embryo chimeras) before any firm conclusion can be drawn, but at this stage it suggests that at least for motor neurons in amphibians there may be a reason for cell death other than simply to eliminate quantitative mismatching of neuron and target populations.

A plausible alternative purpose for cell death is that it is a means of eliminating qualitative errors rather than, or as well as, quantitative errors in pre- and post-synaptic connections. The evidence that this might be so consists of several clear instances where labelling neurons with tracers has revealed connections in the developing animal which are not present in the adult and which are removed by the death of the neurons making them (fig. IV.3).

Fig. IV.3. Connection errors (shown as dotted lines) which are removed by cell death. (*a*) Ectopic and ipsilateral connections from isthmo-optic nuclei to the retina in chick embryos. (*b*) Ipsilateral projections from nasal retina in neonatal rats. (*c*) Inappropriate motor projections in tadpoles.

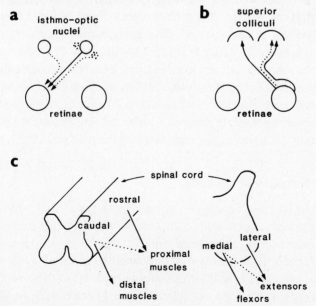

First, in the chick embryo HRP injected into the eye revealed that axons projecting to the retina arise initially not only from the appropriate contralateral isthmo-optic nucleus, but also from ectopic neurons and neurons in the ipsilateral nucleus (fig. IV.3*a*). Most of the ectopic neurons, and all of the ipsilateral neurons, are removed by cell death (Clarke & Cowan, 1976). Secondly, in neonatal rats there are erroneous projections from nasal retina to the ipsilateral superior colliculus. Using a technique of double labelling Jeffery & Perry (1982) were able to show that these projections are removed by cell death (fig. IV.3*b*). Thirdly, in tadpoles different motor neurons and limb muscles arise at different times and there are initially inappropriate connections between them. These connections were detected following retrograde transport of HRP injected into the leg musculature, and it was found that labelled cells establishing connections with the wrong muscles were subsequently eliminated (Lamb, 1977) (fig. IV.3*c*). (See 'Note added in proof', p. 69.)

These examples show that cell death can remove neural connections that are not present in the adult, but it must be pointed out that the proportion of cells making these clearly incorrect connections is small, and certainly less than the proportion which eventually dies. For example in chick limbs we have seen (chapter III.2) that guidance mechanisms deliver motor axons accurately to their targets with at most 10% of axons contacting incorrect muscles, yet about 60% of the motor neurons die. Thus if the only cause of cell death were errors in the pattern of post-synaptic connections, it would be necessary to postulate that additional positional errors occurring within a single muscle are present. These have recently been detected (Bennett & Lavidis, 1982). In addition incorrect *pre*-synaptic connections might reduce the probability of survival for some neurons. The death of some neurons with initially correct pre- and post-synaptic connections might also be accounted for by the subsequent loss of essential inputs or targets through cell death elsewhere in the neuronal network. Mechanisms that could produce the death of neurons with insufficient or erroneous pre- or post-synaptic connections are considered in the next section.

Mechanism of cell death

The fact that neurons do not survive in the animal if their target tissue is removed suggests that an interaction with the target is essential for neuronal survival. A dependence on the target is also apparent when embryonic neurons are grown in culture, since in general neuronal survival is enhanced by supplementing the culture medium with some form of extract of the nerve's target or a related tissue. Thus extracts of embryonic muscle or supernatants of muscle cultures enhance survival of motor neurons (Bennett, Lai & Nurcombe, 1980), extracts of the ciliary body enhance the survival of the parasympathetic ciliary ganglion (Nishi & Berg, 1979) and medium conditioned over cultures of tectum promotes the survival of retinal ganglion cells (Nurcombe & Bennett, 1981). Survival of neurons of sympathetic and sensory ganglia in culture is enhanced by Nerve Growth Factor (NGF), a protein which was first isolated from a mouse sarcoma following observation of its growth-stimulatory effects on sympathetic ganglia in chick embryos (see Levi-Montalcini & Calissano, 1979). NGF was subsequently found in a range of tissues and body fluids (reviewed by Thoenen & Barde, 1980), including a sympathetic target tissue *in vitro* (Ebendal *et al.*, 1980).

Factors other than NGF in heart- and glia-conditioned media can also enhance the survival of sympathetic and sensory neurons in cultures, so there may be subpopulations of ganglion cells with different or changing requirements for growth factors (Barde, Edgar & Thoenen, 1980; Edgar, Barde & Thoenen, 1981). However, the evidence that NGF is obligatory for the survival of sympathetic and sensory neurons in the animal is very strong. NGF injected into neonatal rats prevents both normal and experimentally induced death in the sympathetic ganglia, and in embryonic chicks it prevents cell death in the dorsal root ganglia (Hamburger, Brunso-Bechtold & Yip, 1981). Moreover, uptake and transport mechanisms specific for NGF exist in sympathetic and sensory axons (see Thoenen & Barde, 1980). The most convincing evidence for a role for NGF in the normal animal, though, is the phenomenon of immunosympathectomy, i.e. the death of all sympathetic ganglion cells, when NGF antiserum is injected into neonatal rats (Levi-Montalcini & Cohen, 1960). Sensory neurons are also killed by exposure to NGF antibodies in the embryo (Johnson *et al.*, 1980). Direct evidence for a role for growth factors promoting survival of other neurons *in vivo* is lacking, but it would seem very likely that neurons throughout the nervous system are dependent for their survival on specific growth factors, and that the target cells of the neurons are a source of such factors.

Further evidence for the involvement of the target in neuronal cell death is provided by experiments on motor innervation of muscle in which muscle activity is modulated by various means. Direct stimulation of the muscle causes more motor neuron death than normal (Oppenheim & Nunez, 1982), while inactivation by the post-synaptic blocking agents curare or α-bungarotoxin or by the presynaptic blocking agent botulinum toxin is an effective means of preventing motor neuron death (Pittman & Oppenheim, 1978; Laing & Prestige, 1978). A start has been made on extending these observations to innervation of sympathetic ganglia, where it has been found that blockade of transmission also causes less death in the preganglionic motor nuclei (Oppenheim, Maderdrut & Wells, 1982). While other explanations are possible, these results are consistent with the idea that inactive target cells produce sufficient growth factor to support all neurons in contact with the target, but that with the onset of innervation and activation less factor is produced and some neurons subsequently die.

The failure of neurons to obtain adequate amounts of target-released growth factors provides an obvious explanation for the death of neurons that are in relative excess compared with their target cells, since there would be competition between the neurons for a limited amount of factor available from the target. It can also explain the death of neurons contacting the wrong targets, if either the axons cannot make or maintain adequate contacts with the incorrect target in order to gain access to the factor, or the factor is unsuitable for the errant neurons. Lack of target-released factors may also be involved in the death of neurons with incorrect or insufficient presynaptic inputs if, for example, these neurons are electrically less active and the uptake or utilisation of target-released factors is modulated by electrical activity. It is also possible that some neurons have a direct metabolic requirement for activity or for substances released by appropriate presynaptic terminals. These possibilities are summarised in fig. IV.4.

Neuronal death in invertebrates

Investigation of neuronal death in several invertebrate species has revealed that the nerve target does not play the same key role that it does in vertebrates. In grasshopper embryos a stereotyped pattern of cell division in the segmental ganglia generates thoracic motor neurons which innervate

Fig. IV.4. Possible factors preventing cell death.

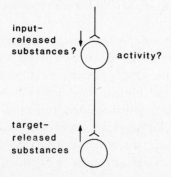

input–
released
substances?   activity?

target–
released
substances

the legs, and homologous neurons in the abdomen which have no tissue to innervate and which die. However, removal of the limb buds does *not* cause the death of those neurons in the thoracic ganglia that would normally innervate leg muscles (Goodman & Bate, 1981). This means that the absence of target tissue is probably not the cause of death of neurons in the abdominal ganglion, but whether there is some other environmental cue or whether the cells are intrinsically specified to die is not known. A similar kind of neuronal death occurs in the nematode, where again there are stereotyped patterns of cell division followed by death of particular, apparently superfluous neurons. The possibility of intrinsically programmed death is suggested by the observation that the neurons die even before they establish processes, but again a local environmental cue cannot be ruled out as yet (Sulston & Horvitz, 1977).

A factor which may be important in the control of neuronal death in some invertebrates is presynaptic input. In the locust visual system a small proportion of neurons in the optic lobe die during normal development. If the retina is prevented from projecting to the optic lobe there is an increased degeneration of optic lobe neurons, whereas an experimentally increased projection produces less cell death (see review by Anderson, Edwards & Palka, 1980). Thus it is likely that some cells in the optic lobe die during normal development because they are not utilised by retinal afferents.

References

Anderson, H., Edwards, J.S. & Palka, J. (1980). Developmental neurobiology of invertebrates. *Annual Review of Neuroscience*, **3**, 97–139.

Barde, Y.-A., Edgar, D. & Thoenen, H. (1980). Sensory neurons in culture: changing requirements for survival factors during embryonic development. *Proceedings of the National Academy of Sciences, USA*, **77**, 1199–203.

Bennett, M.R., Lai, K. & Nurcombe, V. (1980). Identification of embryonic motoneurons *in vitro*: their survival is dependent on skeletal muscle. *Brain Research*, **190**, 537–42.

Bennett, M.R. & Lavidis, N.A. (1982). Development of the topographical projection of motor neurons to amphibian muscle accompanies motor neuron death. *Developmental Brain Research*, **2**, 448–52.

Clarke, P.G.H. (1981). Chance, repetition and error in the development of the nervous system. *Perspectives in Biology and Medicine*, **25**, 2–19.

Clarke, P.G.H. & Cowan, W.M. (1976). The development of the isthmo-optic tract in the chick, with special reference to the occurrence and correction of developmental errors in the location and connections of isthmo-optic neurons. *Journal of Comparative Neurology*, **167**, 143–64.

Cowan, W.M. (1973). Neuronal death as a regulative mechanism in the control of cell number in the nervous system. In *Development and Aging in the Nervous System*, ed. M. Rockstein, pp. 19–41. New York & London: Academic Press.

Ebendal, T., Olson, L., Seiger, A. & Hedlund, K.-O. (1980). Nerve growth factors in the rat iris. *Nature, London*, **286**, 25–8.

Edgar, D., Barde, Y.-A. & Thoenen, H. (1981). Subpopulations of cultured chick sympathetic neurons differ in their requirements for survival factors. *Nature, London*, **289**, 244–5.

Goodman, C.S. & Bate, M. (1981). Neuronal development in the grasshopper. *Trends in Neurosciences*, **4**, 163–9.

Hamburger, V. (1980). Trophic interactions in neurogenesis: a personal historical account. *Annual Review of Neuroscience*, **3**, 269–78.

Hamburger, V., Brunso-Bechtold, J.L. & Yip, J.W. (1981). Neuronal death in the spinal ganglia of the chick embryo and its reduction by nerve growth factor. *Journal of Neuroscience*, **1**, 60–71.

Hamburger, V. & Levi-Montalcini, R. (1949). Proliferation, differentiation and degeneration in the spinal ganglia of the chick embryo under normal and experimental conditions. *Journal of Experimental Zoology*, **111**, 457–507.

Hamburger, V. & Oppenheim, R.W. (1982). Naturally occurring neuronal death in vertebrates. *Neuroscience Commentaries*, **1**, 39–55.

Hollyday, M. & Hamburger, V. (1976). Reduction in naturally occurring motor neuron loss by enlargement of the periphery. *Journal of Comparative Neurology*, **170**, 311–20.

Jeffery, G. & Perry, V.H. (1982). Evidence for ganglion-cell death during development of the ipsilateral retinal projection in the rat. *Developmental Brain Research*, **2**, 176–80.

Johnson, E.M., Gorin, P.D., Brandeis, L.D. & Pearson, J. (1980). Dorsal root ganglion neurons are destroyed by exposure *in utero* to maternal antibody to nerve growth factor. *Science*, **210**, 916–18.

Laing, N.G. & Prestige, M.C. (1978). Prevention of spontaneous motoneurone death in chick embryos. *Journal of Physiology*, **282**, 33P.

Lamb, A.H. (1976). The projection patterns of the ventral horn to the hind limb during development. *Developmental Biology*, **54**, 82–99.

Lamb, A.H. (1977). Neuronal death in the development of the somatotopic projections of the ventral horn in *Xenopus*. *Brain Research*, **134**, 145–50.

Lamb, A.H. (1980). Motoneurone counts in *Xenopus* frogs reared with one bilaterally-innervated hind limb. *Nature, London*, **284**, 347–50.

Landmesser, L. & Pilar, G. (1976). Fate of ganglionic synapses and ganglion cell axons during normal and induced cell death. *Journal of Cell Biology*, **68**, 357–74.

Levi-Montalcini, R. & Calissano, P. (1979). The Nerve Growth Factor. *Scientific American*, **240** (June), 44–53.

Levi-Montalcini, R. & Cohen, S. (1960). Effects of the extract of the mouse submaxillary salivary glands on the sympathetic system of mammals. *Annals of the New York Academy of Sciences*, **85**, 324–41.

Linden, R. & Perry, V.H. (1982). Ganglion-cell death within the developing retina: a regulatory role for retinal dendrites? *Neuroscience*, **7**, 2813–27.

Nishi, R. & Berg, D.K. (1979). Survival and development of ciliary ganglion neurons grown alone in cell culture. *Nature, London*, **277**, 232–4.

Nurcombe, V. & Bennett, M.R. (1981). Embryonic chick retinal ganglion cells identified 'in vitro'. Their survival is dependent on a factor from the optic tectum. *Experimental Brain Research*, **44**, 249–58.

Okada, N. & Oppenheim, R.W. (1981). *Society for Neuroscience Abstracts*, **7**, 291.

Oppenheim, R.W., Maderdrut, J.L. & Wells, D.J. (1982). Reduction of naturally-occurring cell death in the thoraco-lumbar preganglionic cell column of the chick embryo by nerve growth factor and hemicholinium-3. *Developmental Brain Research*, **3**, 134–9.

Oppenheim, R.W. & Nunez, R. (1982). Electrical stimulation of hind limb increases neuronal cell death in chick embryo. *Nature, London*, **295**, 57–9.

Pittman, R.H. & Oppenheim, R.W. (1978). Neuromuscular blockade increases motoneuron survival during normal cell death in chick embryo. *Nature, London*, **271**, 364–6.

Shieh, P. (1951). The neoformation of cells of preganglionic type in the cervical spinal cord of the chick embryo following its transplantation to the thoracic level. *Journal of Experimental Zoology*, **117**, 354–95.

Sulston, J.E. & Horvitz, H.R. (1977). Post-embryonic cell lineages in the nematode, *Caenorhabditis elegans*. *Developmental Biology*, **56**, 110–56.

Thoenen, H. & Barde, T.-A. (1980). Physiology of Nerve Growth Factor. *Physiological Reviews*, **60**, 1284–335.

Note added in proof
It is now apparent that while ipsilaterally projecting neurons within the isthmo-optic nucleus *may* be selectively eliminated by cell death, the ectopic neurons are *not* (O'Leary & Cowan (1982) *Journal of Comparative Neurology*, **212**, 399–416).

IV.2

Excess connections and their elimination

Cajal and his associates, in the early part of this century, were the first to present evidence that there might be an initial excess of connections in the developing nervous system. In CNS tissue stained by the Golgi method it was apparent that many more spines were present on the dendrites of some neurons during development than in the adult. It was also noticed that muscle fibres in neonatal animals appeared to be contacted by branches of several axons, in contrast to adult fibres, which were innervated invariably by a single axon. Further research on this phenomenon awaited its rediscovery more than 50 years later, when physiological investigations of neonatal muscles revealed that individual muscle fibres were innervated initially by more than one axon. It has since been shown that elimination of the excess inputs requires activity in the muscle. The mechanism of this elimination may involve competition between the separate inputs for a muscle-released growth factor.

A similar excess of presynaptic inputs in neonatal animals has also been demonstrated physiologically on neurons of autonomic ganglia and on Purkinje cells of the cerebellum. Direct visualisation of these excess inputs has so far not been possible, but at many other places in the CNS axon branching can be seen to be initially more diffuse than in the mature nervous system. The most well-known examples are from loci in the visual system, in particular the lateral geniculate nucleus, the superior colliculus and layer IV of the visual cortex, where the axon terminals corresponding to each eye are in discrete bands in the adult but are intermingled in embryonic or neonatal animals. Cortical neurons in the neonate have also been shown to have axon collaterals projecting to the contralateral cortex or entering the pyramidal tract, and many of these collaterals are not present in the adult. It is important to note that in all these cases the phase of cell death for the presynaptic neurons is over before the excess presynaptic inputs are eliminated. It follows that the excess inputs are a consequence of diffuse branching of the presynaptic axons rather than a consequence of an excess of presynaptic neurons, and that the elimination of the excess inputs is brought about by a remodelling of the axon branches.

Another much studied example of synapse reorganisation concerns the connections that relay visual information from layer IV to the other layers in the visual cortex. Diffuse branching of the axons that project from layer IV has not been visualised directly, but its presence can be inferred from the receptive fields of the neurons, that is from the visual stimuli that make the neurons respond. Initially the neurons respond to a wider range of visual stimuli than they do in the adult, but a fine tuning to specific stimuli gradually develops partly as a result of visual experience during a certain 'critical' period. Abnormal visual experience during this time produces correspondingly abnormal receptive fields, which become permanent by the end of the critical period. The modifications may be achieved by functional suppression of some inputs, as well as by the elimination of axon branches.

Other examples of critical periods that may have excess connections as their basis are given in the final section of this chapter.

Multiple innervation at the neuromuscular junction

The presence of more than one functional input at the neuromuscular junction of neonatal muscle fibres was first detected by Redfern, who was recording *in vitro* from muscle fibres in which the end-plate potentials had been reduced to subthreshold levels with bath-applied curare. Under such conditions the end-plate potential of an adult muscle fibre has a relatively constant amplitude, but in the neonate end-plate potentials of individual fibres show several consistent stepwise increments as more axons are stimulated in the muscle nerve (Redfern, 1970). The presence of excess axonal branches was confirmed by demonstrations that individual motor units were several times larger than in the adult (Bagust, Lewis & Westerman, 1973; Brown, Jansen & Van Essen, 1976), and by visualisation of intramuscular nerves and nerve terminals in the light and electron microscopes (Riley, 1976; Korneliussen & Jansen, 1976).

Interest has now centred on explaining how all axonal branches except one are eliminated from the neuromuscular junction. As with neuronal death, the precise nature of the mechanism has not been established unequivocally, but a number of conclusions about the elimination process have been made: it occurs by retraction rather than degeneration of branches; it appears to depend on competition between axons for muscle fibres, and in particular for something at the post-synaptic site; and the competition is modulated by post-synaptic activity. The evidence for these conclusions is discussed below.

Eliminated inputs are retracted. It was originally thought that the excess inputs at the neuromuscular junction were removed by degeneration (Rosenthal & Taraskevich, 1977). More careful analysis showed that any nerve degeneration seen in the neonatal muscles was insufficient to account for the removal of the excess branches (Bixby, 1981). Retraction bulbs can be seen in the light microscope during the elimination period (Riley, 1977), and in the electron microscope it is clear that axonal structural components are being resorbed at such structures (Riley, 1981). The structural components are presumably redistributed to surviving branches.

Axons compete for muscle cells. The fact that in mammalian muscles elimination of excess axonal inputs proceeds until exactly one axon remains in contact with each muscle fibre has given rise to the idea of a *competitive interaction* between the nerve terminals for occupancy of muscle fibres. If instead of competing for muscle fibres neurons simply lost at random a proportion of their terminals, this would lead to complete denervation of some muscle fibres and permanent multiple innervation of others, neither of which occurs in normal mammalian muscles (Brown *et al.*, 1976). A diffuse competition between neurons for or against occupancy of the muscle in general can also be excluded since this too could not lead to muscle fibres innervated invariably by a single axon. The competition that exists between nerves must therefore be related to occupancy of individual muscle fibres.

That normal elimination requires competition from other axons can be tested by removing some of the competing axons and observing whether there is a failure of branch loss from remaining axons. If neonatal rat muscles are partly denervated at birth and then allowed to mature, the motor units end up somewhat larger than in the normal adult, but apparently somewhat smaller than at the time of the partial denervation. These observations were taken as evidence for an 'intrinsic tendency' of some terminals to withdraw (Thompson & Jansen, 1977), but it is also clear that if there is such a tendency it cannot on its own reduce the motor units to normal adult size.

Competition that results in a reduction in synaptic effectiveness, but not necessarily complete elimination, has been demonstrated between two foreign nerves implanted onto a denervated muscle in adult frogs. Transmission at individual synapses on fibres which are innervated by both nerves is less effective than on fibres which receive inputs from only one nerve (Grinnell, Letinsky & Rheuben, 1979). The competition is probably mediated by action potentials in the muscle fibres (see below).

The post-synaptic site maintains axon branches. During the elimination of excess synapses, histological estimates of the proportion of multiply innervated fibres do not exceed estimates obtained by the method of graded stimulation and intracellular recording (see Brown, Holland & Hopkins, 1981*a*). This implies that terminal branches are withdrawn at or near the time they lose functional contact with muscle fibres, and it suggests that adequate contact with a muscle fibre at the end-plate is required to stabilise a terminal axon branch. The property of the post-synaptic membrane that could maintain survival of axon branches remains to be determined. It may be a substance in the extracellular matrix of the end-plate which influences nerve terminal growth by a contact interaction, or it may be a diffusible growth factor released from the junctional membrane (possibly identical to that for which whole neurons are thought to compete for their survival earlier in development). The latter possibility is supported by the observation that locally applied NGF can promote survival of individual sympathetic nerve branches in tissue culture (Campenot, 1977).

Post-synaptic activity modulates the competition. The normal elimination of excess axonal branches at the neuromuscular junction is accelerated by direct muscle stimulation (O'Brien, Ostberg & Vrbova, 1978) and is slowed or prevented by relative inactivity brought about by tenotomy (Benoit & Changeux, 1975), or transmission blockade with botulinum toxin (Brown *et al.*, 1981*b*) or α-bungarotoxin (Duxson, 1982). Muscle activity also modulates the elimination of multiple innervation that follows the ectopic innervation of denervated muscle fibres by an implanted foreign nerve. The foreign nerve initially makes end-plates spaced at random along individual fibres, and activity is required to eliminate these (Lømo & Slater, 1980). There appears to be a selective elimination of closely spaced inputs (Kuffler, Thompson & Jansen, 1980) and a similar effect is seen for the elimination of post-synaptic specialisations if the foreign nerve is cut and the muscle is stimulated directly (T. Lømo, S. Pockett & H. Sommerschild, unpublished). This apparent distance-dependent effect may reflect a limited capacity of the active muscle fibres to maintain post-synaptic specialisations along a given length of fibre. A similar conclusion was suggested by the observation that paralysis of chick embryos with curare produces regularly spaced synapses on muscle fibres that would normally be singly innervated, and decreases the spacing between synapses on multiply innervated fibres (Gordon *et al.*, 1974). Direct stimulation of the nerves to developing embryonic chick hindlimb muscles can also alter the pattern of innervation: a 'slow' pattern of activity (continuous stimulation at 0.5 hertz: see also chapter IV.4, p. 106) produces multiple synaptic sites on muscle fibres that would normally be singly innervated (Toutant *et al.*, 1980). Thus the pattern of activation appears to determine which muscle fibres develop and retain into adulthood a distributed multiple innervation.

It remains to be established how post-synaptic activity regulates axon branch survival. Some authors have postulated the existence of a muscle-released proteolytic enzyme that digests axon terminals and that might be released in smaller quantities when fibres are inactive (O'Brien, Ostberg & Vrbova, 1980). It is perhaps more likely that activity affects the synthesis, release or degradation of a substance that maintains survival of axon branches on muscle fibres.

Fig. IV.5 summarises the available observations on synapse elimination at the neuromuscular junction by illustrating schematically the gradual loss of

Fig. IV.5. Model for activity-modulated neuronal competition at the motor end-plate. Amount and distribution of nerve terminal survival factor associated with a given muscle fibre is indicated by plus signs. Amount and direction of supply of materials from cell body is indicated by open arrows. (*a*) Muscle fibre is initially very 'innervatible'. (*b*) Activity after functional contact (here by two axons) reduces 'innervatibility' to a single site. (*c*) Activity may further reduce the availability of the growth/survival factor from the muscle. Solid arrows indicate that the terminal with the greater amount of contact with the post-synaptic site gains enhanced supply and so grows by positive feedback. Similarly the smaller terminal shrinks. (*d*) The terminal which loses all contact with the muscle is immediately withdrawn.

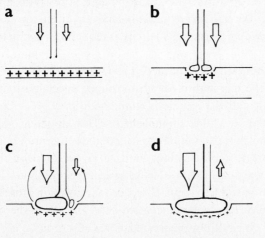

attractiveness of the end-plate brought about by post-synaptic activity, and the withdrawal of axons that lose contact with the end-plate. If it is assumed that increased contact with the end-plate increases axon branch survival, positive feedback could stabilise a larger terminal and destabilise a smaller terminal, and this could lead to the elimination of some terminals (Purves & Lichtman, 1980). The effectiveness of the feedback would have to be very great to explain why one and only one terminal invariably survives at each end-plate, so it is possible that some important aspect of synapse elimination at the neuromuscular junction has yet to be identified. It will be seen later in this chapter that correlated pre- and post-synaptic activity may play an important role in stabilising synapses in the CNS. While there is as yet no evidence for this at the neuromuscular junction an interaction of this nature may be necessary to prevent the last remaining nerve terminal from eliminating itself.

Excess presynaptic inputs in ganglia and the cerebellum

Excess functional synapses in autonomic ganglia and in the cerebellum have been demonstrated physiologically with the technique of graded stimulation of presynaptic axons and intracellular recording from post-synaptic cells. Much less is known about the probable mechanisms for the elimination of excess synapses at these sites compared with those in muscle.

In the neonatal rat the cells of the submandibular ganglion are functionally innervated by up to five preganglionic fibres, but by 40 days of age the adult state of one input per ganglion cell is established (fig. IV.6). When the synaptic boutons of the preganglionic axons were stained and counted in the light microscope, it was apparent that the total number of boutons on the cells increased throughout the period that the number of inputs from different preganglionic axons on each cell was declining. This

Fig. IV.6. Elimination of multiple innervation in the submandibular ganglion of the rat.

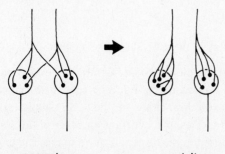

neonate   adult

implies that elimination of some inputs allows redistribution and concentration of each preganglionic axon on fewer ganglion cells (Lichtman, 1977).

Neurons in the guinea-pig superior cervical ganglion, which in the adult are innervated by six or seven separate preganglionic axons, have nearly twice as many axonal inputs in the immature animal. The inputs in the neonate arise from an average of four contiguous spinal cord segmental levels, whereas in the adult they arise from less than three (Lichtman & Purves, 1980). Thus it is possible that graded segmental labels are involved in the competitive removal of excess inputs from ganglion cells.

In the rabbit ciliary ganglion the post-synaptic cells are contacted initially by four or five axons, but in the adult this is reduced to a range of one to five. There is a strong correlation between the number of inputs and the number of dendrites possessed by the adult but not by the neonatal ganglion cells, suggesting that the separate inputs are segregated onto separate dendrites during development. Thus competition for separate dendrites rather than for an entire neuron may allow multiple inputs to survive on adult nerve cells (Hume & Purves, 1981). Nothing is known as yet about the mechanism of such dendritic competition, but it is possible that pre- and post-synaptic activity is involved.

In the CNS only one example of excess innervation has been detected directly by physiological means. The Purkinje cells in the adult rat cerebellum are innervated by one climbing fibre from the inferior olive, but in the neonate two or three climbing fibre inputs can be detected. In the adult the synapses of each climbing fibre are located on the dendrites, but in the neonate synapses also occur on the cell body (Crepel, Mariani & Delhaye-Bouchaud, 1976). The multiple climbing fibre inputs persist in various cerebellar mouse mutants and experimental animals that have in common a failure in the formation of parallel fibre synapses on the Purkinje dendrites. It has been suggested that the parallel fibre synapses may strengthen the competitive interaction among the climbing fibres by decreasing their supply of some trophic factor from the Purkinje cells (Crepel, 1982).

Diffuse connections in the central nervous system

Although direct physiological demonstration of excess presynaptic inputs in the CNS is limited to the Purkinje cells in the cerebellum, histological studies of axon branching in the CNS suggest that the phenomenon is likely to be widespread. A transient stage of diffuse axonal branching has been visualised in the terminations of axons relaying visual information at several sites in the brain, and axonal branches which are eliminated as the animal matures have now also been found in the pyramidal tract and in the corpus callosum.

Several histological methods have been used to delineate the axon branching in the visual pathways, but the most successful has been autoradiography. A radioactively labelled amino acid is injected into one eye from where it is transported along the axons of the retinal ganglion cells to their terminals in the lateral geniculate nucleus (LGN) and superior colliculus; subsequent autoradiography of sections of the brain can then reveal the gross distribution of the terminals from one eye in these two areas. Some label is also transferred to the cells in the LGN and thence to the terminals of these cells in layer IV of the visual cortex, where it can also be detected by so-called transneuronal autoradiography. If one eye is injected in the adult the terminals in the LGN, superior colliculus and visual cortex are revealed as discrete bands of label interdigitated with equal-sized unlabelled bands corresponding to the uninjected eye (fig. IV.8). During development, however, the terminals are initially inter-mingled, and gradually segregate into bands – by birth in the LGN and superior colliculus and by several weeks of age in the visual cortex (Rakic, 1977). By recording from neurons in layer IV it is possible to demonstrate that there is a correlated functional segregation of the inputs from each eye (Hubel, Wiesel & Le Vay, 1977), and selective staining of terminal arborisations of individual geniculate afferents in the cortex has also verified the loss of branches in the regions corresponding to the bands of the other eye (fig. IV.7) (see Wiesel, 1982).

Experiments similar to those performed on neonatal muscles indicate that the segregation into bands is dependent on competition between terminals of the left and right eyes. If one eye is removed in the embryo the terminals of the other eye do not condense into bands (Rakic, 1981). Activity seems to be important, because if both eyes are sutured shut at birth the separation of the geniculate afferents into bands in layer IV is

Fig. IV.7. Terminal branching of an afferent from the lateral geniculate nucleus to layer IV in the visual cortex of the neonate and of the adult monkey.

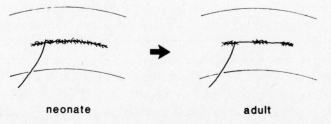

neonate   **adult**

reduced (Swindale, 1981). Moreover if only one eye is sutured shut at birth, its bands in layer IV shrink while those of the open eye remain wider than normal, suggesting that the more active open eye has a competitive advantage over the closed eye.

Further insight into the competitive interaction between the eyes has come from observations on bands in the amphibian tectum. In amphibians the decussation of axons from each eye is complete so there is normally no possibility of alternate banding of retinal afferents on the tectum. However, bands remarkably similar to those in the mammalian colliculus or visual cortex can be induced in the tectum if it receives projections from both eyes (Levine & Jacobson, 1975) or from a transplanted third eye (Law & Constantine-Paton, 1981). Similar bands develop if a double-nasal or double-temporal compound eye projects to the tectum, and it has been suggested that the bands develop when the normal guidance or recognition mechanism which distributes terminals across the target in a retinotopic fashion combines with some 'nearest-neighbour' interaction between axons favouring local segregation of terminals from the same eye (Fawcett & Willshaw, 1982). One of the properties that neighbouring retinal ganglion cells share is relative synchrony of their activity, and activity is involved in the nearest-neighbour interactions because bands do not form in a tectum receiving projections from eyes rendered electrically silent by injections of tetrodotoxin (Meyer, 1982). Moreover, post-synaptic activity seems to be important for stabilising retinal axon terminals, because the terminals vacate a small area of tectum that has been blocked post-synaptically with α-bungarotoxin and make new connections nearby (Freeman, 1977). The basis of the nearest-neighbour interaction may therefore be synchronous activity in axon terminals and post-synaptic tectal cells, producing stabilisation of connections in localised bands. The randomised pattern of bands in the mammalian colliculus and cortex could develop in the same way, but in the LGN, where the bands are always in the same places, some additional guidance or recognition mechanism must operate on the axons from each eye.

The most recent reports of diffuse connections in the CNS concern wholly aberrant collaterals rather than simply excess terminal branches. The presence of these collaterals is inferred from the fact that dyes injected into a given part of the brain of neonates can be detected subsequently in cell bodies at another site, whereas these cells are not labelled by an injection in the more mature animal. The axon collaterals which presumably pick up the dye are not removed by cell death because the labelled cell bodies are still present weeks or months later. Thus an injection of dye into the pyramidal tract of newborn rats labels neurons right across the cortex, but in 3-week-old rats injections do not label visual cortical neurons (Stanfield, O'Leary & Fricks, 1982). Similarly injections of dye into the cortex of newborn cats label cells widely in the corresponding region of the contralateral cortex via collaterals in the corpus callosum, whereas in adult cats the connections are more restricted in somatosensory areas (O'Leary, Stanfield & Cowan, 1981), and in visual areas corresponding to the midline in visual space (Innocenti, 1981). It is interesting that in cats with a natural or artificially induced squint (strabismus) there are considerably more connections between the visual areas (Lund, Mitchell & Henry, 1978), which is consistent with the possibility of a retention of callosal collaterals joining areas that share the same region of visual space and so are activated synchronously by visual stimuli. A similar mechanism in frogs probably maintains connections that link areas of left and right tecta that correspond to the region of overlap of the visual fields of each eye (Keating, 1974).

Modification of receptive fields in the visual cortex

Visual information is delivered to the neurons of layer IV of the visual cortex by the geniculate afferents and is then distributed to the other layers by intracortical connections. The pattern of these connections, and the changes that occur in them during development, have not been visualised directly but have been inferred from the changes in the visual stimuli that activate the neurons, that is from changes in the receptive field properties of the neurons.

The knowledge of the properties of the neurons of the visual pathway is due largely to the work of Hubel and Wiesel, which will be summarised briefly here (for more detailed overview see Hubel & Wiesel, 1979, or Hubel, 1982). The receptive field of a neuron in the visual pathway is determined by the convergence of inputs from lower-order neurons (fig. IV.8). Ganglion cells of the retina integrate the output of photoreceptors and respond to changes in light intensity in small circular patches of visual space. Neurons of the LGN and of layer IV have similar receptive fields and hence probably act mainly as relays for axons from the retina. Convergence is evident beyond layer IV, where neurons will usually respond only to stimuli with straight edges of a specific orientation moving in a specific small area of visual space. Neurons with similar orientation specificities are distributed across the cortex in regular 'columns' or more accurately 'slabs'. Neighbouring slabs have slightly different orientation preferences or specificities, so that in a direction normal to the slabs a full 360 of orientation specificities is encountered across a distance of several milli-metres. Most neurons have inputs from both eyes, and one of the interesting features of such binocular neurons is that the receptive field properties in each eye are very similar. One eye usually dominates or drives a binocular neuron more effectively than the other, and neurons with similar ocular dominance are organised in an independent pattern of columns which reflects the underlying bands of afferents in layer IV.

The binocularity of cortical neurons was the first property found to be modifiable by experience. Hubel & Wiesel (1970) discovered that closing one eye of kittens for a few days or more during a 'critical period' of 4–8 weeks of age caused a marked reduction in the number of binocularly driven cells in the cortex. However, closure of one eye also causes shrinkage of its afferents in layer IV, so it was not clear whether the loss of binocularity of higher-order neurons was a consequence of this shrinkage or of a more direct effect on the intracortical connections. Loss of binocularity was also noted in cats that had been raised with an artificial squint (strabismus) following removal of one of the extraocular muscles, and the same effect was achieved when kittens were reared with daily

Fig. IV.8. Pattern of connections to the normal mammalian visual cortex. Above: convergence of inputs from each eye to produce binocular receptive fields in neurons beyond layer IV of the visual cortex. Convergence of many inputs produces the other receptive field properties of cortical neurons. LGN, lateral geniculate nucleus. Below left: pattern of banding of afferents from left and right eyes in layer IV. Below right: pattern of orientation slabs above and below layer IV.

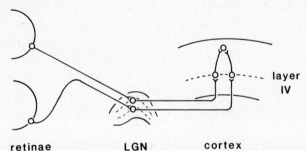

retinae   LGN   cortex

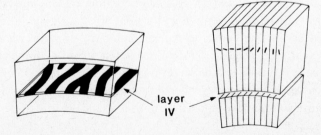

layer
IV

alternate occlusion of each eye throughout the critical period (Hubel & Wiesel, 1965). In both these cases there was no relative reduction in the cortical drive from either eye because the frequencies of purely monocular cells driven by each eye were usually similar. This meant that the loss of binocularity could be ascribed to a direct effect of the experimental manipulations on connections from the bands of layer IV that would normally converge to produce binocular neurons. The loss of binocularity can be attributed to asynchrony in activity in adjacent bands even in those animals with squint: in a normal animal natural stimuli activate similar regions of each retina synchronously and hence adjacent afferent terminations in the cortex are synchronously active; in animals with a squint the synchronously active inputs from each eye are separated on the cortex, and adjacent bands are therefore asynchronous.

The orientation preference of cortical neurons has also been shown to be modified by experience. If kittens are reared with their vision restricted to contours of one orientation, then their cortical cells will respond only to contours of that orientation. Again the modifications can be made only during a critical period of between 4 and 8 weeks of age (e.g. Blakemore & Mitchell, 1973).

Given that abnormal visual experience can produce these changes in cortical circuitry, it is natural to ask whether normal visual experience plays some part in establishing normal response properties in cortical cells. The first observations on the properties of visual cortical neurons in normal young kittens gave the impression that all properties were innately determined (Hubel & Wiesel, 1963), which made their modifiability seem superfluous and potentially disadvantageous. However, it is now clear that the properties are only partly specified in visually naive animals. In the kitten, receptive field sizes are larger than in the adult, orientation specificities are poorly defined or broadly tuned, and in binocular cells there is poor concordance between the receptive field properties for each eye (Pettigrew, 1974). In the monkey, some properties may be more accurately prespecified than in kittens (Wiesel & Hubel, 1974), but a rigorous study of orientation specificity and binocular receptive fields in the neonatal monkey is lacking (Pettigrew, 1978). The critical period can therefore be seen as a time when cortical connections are modifiable and when the response properties resulting from the connections can be 'fine-tuned' by visual experience.

The cellular mechanism underlying the experience-induced changes in cortical connections is as yet unknown, but as with the modifications in muscle, certain aspects of the mechanism have emerged from the large number of experiments that have been performed. These are summarised briefly below:

Role of activity. In kittens deprived of all visual experience, the responses of the neurons do not sharpen up but instead gradually deteriorate. Eventually a high proportion of neurons fails to respond to any visual stimulation, suggesting that connections which are not reinforced by activity are lost. If, on the other hand, vision is restricted to contours of a single orientation, then in the adult there are many more cells responding specifically to that orientation than there would normally be, the orientation columns in the cortex are wider and there are few non-responsive cells (e.g. Rauschecker & Singer, 1981). Exposure to a single contour therefore 'rescues' not only those neurons that would respond to that orientation in the normal adult, but also additional adjacent neurons. In the neonate these extra neurons would presumably be active in response to the stimulus because of the broad tuning of receptive fields.

The fine tuning can occur with very little experience. Kittens reared in the dark need only be exposed to a restricted visual environment for an hour during the critical period to produce restricted responses in the cortical cells (Blakemore & Mitchell, 1973). Responses can even be specified in an anaesthetised visually naive kitten in several minutes during the testing of a neuron's receptive field (Pettigrew, Olson & Barlow, 1973).

Competition between inputs. Another feature of tuning is the competition between inputs subserving different orientations. Normal experience consists of exposure to contours of all possible orientations, but this does not maintain broad tuning of cortical cells, nor does it produce cells responding to several discrete orientations. Instead inputs to cortical cells compete until only one sharply tuned orientation succeeds in activating each cell. A similar competition occurs between inputs from each eye, ensuring that the receptive field properties are identical in each eye.

The degree of synchrony required to reinforce connections for the maintenance of binocularity has been analysed using several methods to produce rapidly alternating occlusion of kittens' eyes (Blasdel & Pettigrew, 1979). It was found that there must be less than 10 seconds between alternate occlusions to maintain normal numbers of binocular cells. The degree of synchrony required to maintain different inputs from the same eye on a cortical cell is presumably similar.

A suitable mechanism invoking activity to achieve this competition between inputs must involve a selective stabilisation or growth of those inputs where there is synchrony of pre- and post-synaptic activity, and a gradual loss of other inputs. Synapse modifications of this nature were suggested originally by Hebb to be the basis of learning and memory.

Stent (1973) suggested that transmitter action at the post-synaptic site might somehow protect the site from being degraded by action potentials induced by the transmitter, but this remains to be verified or refuted. Target-released nerve growth factors could be involved in the stabilisation of synapses if their release and uptake are linked with post- and presynaptic activity.

Role of noradrenaline. Modifiability of ocular dominance on cortical cells appears to require the presence of noradrenaline in the cortex. This was discovered when destruction of the adrenergic projections to the cortex by 6-hydroxydopamine at the onset of the critical period prevented the changes in dominance induced by monocular occlusion. Plasticity is restored in the vicinity of a cannula releasing noradrenaline onto the cortical surface (Kasamatsu, Pettigrew & Ary, 1979). The noradrenaline may act in a relatively non-specific way by increasing the excitability of cortical neurons and thereby gating all post-synaptic activity.

Synaptogenesis and synapse elimination. Morphometric analysis of the visual cortex of monkeys has revealed that the absolute number of synapses in the visual cortex increases until 6 months of age (O'Kusky & Colonnier, 1982), and there is a similar increase in the number of dendritic spines (Lund, Boothe & Lund, 1977). It is not known whether this period of growth represents a strengthening of immature synapses that escape detection in the early post-natal period, or whether visual experience stimulates growth of axons and dendrites to the extent that wholly new axon–target cell connections form. After 6 months of age the number of synapses declines by approximately 50% and dendrites similarly lose complexity, so it is clear that synapse elimination does indeed occur as the visual system matures.

Functional suppression of synapses. Although much of the fine tuning is likely to be achieved by withdrawal of excess branches, certain experimental procedures can produce a rapid restoration of some inputs, which is consistent with derepression of functionally suppressed synapses rather than a physical regrowth. Thus cortical drive from a deprived eye is enhanced immediately following removal of the other eye (Kratz, Spear & Smith, 1976), stimulation of a deprived eye with rotating gratings produces a rapid enhancement of its input to cortical cells (Martin *et al.*, 1979), and increasing cortical excitability with bicuculline (an antagonist of the inhibitory transmitter γ-aminobutyric acid) unmasks additional inputs to cortical cells (Sillito, 1975; Duffy *et al.*, 1976).

Little is known about the loss of modifiability which marks the end of the critical period. Myelination of axons has been suggested as one factor that could prevent retraction or regrowth of axon branches of afferents in layer IV, and possibly of higher-order neurons. Other possibilities include loss of ability of pre- and post-synaptic cells to make new synapses and irreversible maturation of synapses. It is possible to prolong the critical period for modification of binocularity by raising kittens in the dark (Cynader & Mitchell, 1980), but this also makes many cortical cells unresponsive to any visual stimulus (see above).

Synaptic reorganisation in other systems

Examples of critical periods for the modification of brain or behaviour are given below. The neuronal basis of these critical periods has not been identified, but it will not be surprising if initially diffuse connections, some of which are strengthened and some of which are eliminated, are found to be involved.

Two examples have been described in the auditory system of birds: sound localisation in owls and the development of song production. Adult barn owls are able to localise accurately sounds in space, but they lose this ability whenever binaural input is distorted with an earplug. Young birds, however, learn to compensate for an earplug (Knudsen, Knudsen & Esterly, 1982). Most songbirds learn their songs during a resticted period in their first year of life. The learning involves modification of the bird's own innate calls until they match other adult calls or other environmental sounds (not necessarily even bird calls). After the critical period no new themes are acquired (Nottebohm, 1970).

An often-cited example of neural modification that is produced only during a critical neonatal period concerns the development of the somatosensory cortex in rodents. In transverse sections of the cortex the normal adult animal has an array of characteristic barrel-shaped structures formed by the neurons associated with the sensory apparatus of single facial vibrissae. Destruction of individual vibrissae in animals a few days old prevents the development of the corresponding barrels, whereas the same injury in the adult is without visible effect (Van der Loos & Woolsey, 1973). It is not clear whether this failure in barrel development is caused simply by the loss of afferent impulses to the cortex or by the degeneration of sensory and higher-order neurons following removal of the sensory target tissue.

The ability of animals to regulate their body temperature is modified by experience during development. If the animals are not exposed to cool temperatures during rearing then their ability to maintain their body temperature in a cool environment is impaired (Cooper, Ferguson & Veale, 1980; Dawson *et al.*, 1982). This effect is not caused by changes in the sensitivity of peripheral thermoreceptors, so a central regulatory modification is likely.

In humans the critical period during which binocular vision can be compromised by strabismus extends up to approximately five years of age (Banks, Aslin & Letson, 1975). Beyond this age the excess connections responsible for binocularity in the visual cortex have presumably been eliminated. Are there excess connections elsewhere in the cortex, and if so, what is the critical period for their modification? It is interesting to consider that in the first few years of life children can assimilate with little effort not just one but many languages, and can develop skills in music and movement that are insuperably difficult for the inexperienced adult. Excess modifiable connections in appropriate regions of the cortex and elsewhere in the brain may be the basis of these remarkable feats of learning.

Conclusion

The essential feature of the stage of synapse reorganisation is that there are excess connections available from which a selection can be made, most probably by some kind of functional validation involving synchronous pre- and post-synaptic activity, possibly coupled with uptake of axon growth factors. Production of some of the excess connections may be deliberate: for example, the collateral branches of cortical neurons probably develop on all neurons of a particular phenotype and grow to the contralateral cortex as part of the general cortical development programme. Diffuse terminal branching, on the other hand, is in some instances probably an inevitable response to growth stimuli when the axons arrive at the uninnervated target.

The critical period most probably corresponds to the time when excess connections are present and modifiable by experience-related neuronal activity. In the adult brain the excess connections that were not used during development are gone, but the mechanisms that led to competition between the connections may still operate on the more limited connections that remain and thus contribute to adult plasticity.

References

Multiple innervation at the neuromuscular junction

Bagust, J., Lewis, D.M. & Westerman, R.A. (1973). Polyneuronal innervation of kitten skeletal muscle. *Journal of Physiology*, **229**, 241–55.

Benoit, P. & Changeux, J.-P. (1975). Consequences of tenotomy on the evolution of multi-innervation in developing rat soleus muscle. *Brain Research*, **99**, 345–58.

Bixby, J.L. (1981). Ultrastructural observations on synapse elimination in neonatal rabbit skeletal muscle. *Journal of Neurocytology*, **10**, 81–100.

Brown, M.C., Holland, R.L. & Hopkins, W.G. (1981*a*). Excess neuronal inputs during development. In *Development in the Nervous System*, ed. D.R. Garrod & J.D. Feldman, pp. 245–62. Cambridge University Press.

Brown, M.C., Holland, R.L. & Hopkins, W.G. (1981*b*). Restoration of focal multiple innervation in rat muscles by transmission block during a critical stage of development. *Journal of Physiology*, **318**, 355–64.

Brown, M.C., Jansen, J.K.S. & Van Essen, D. (1976). Polyneuronal innervation of skeletal muscle in new-born rats and its elimination during maturation. *Journal of Physiology*, **261**, 387–442.

Campenot, R.B. (1977). Local control of neurite development by nerve growth factor. *Proceedings of the National Academy of Sciences, USA*, **74**, 4516–19.

Duxson, M.J. (1982). The effect of post-synaptic block on development of the neuromuscular junction in postnatal rats. *Journal of Neurocytology*, **11**, 395–408.

Gordon, T., Perry, R., Tuffery, A.R. & Vrbova, G. (1974). Possible mechanisms determining synapse formation in developing skeletal muscles of the chick. *Cell and Tissue Research*, **155**, 13–25.

Grinnell, A.D., Letinsky, M.S. & Rheuben, M.B. (1979). Competitive interaction between foreign nerves innervating frog skeletal muscle. *Journal of Physiology*, **289**, 241–62.

Korneliussen, H. & Jansen, J.K.S. (1976). Morphological aspects of the elimination of polyneuronal innervation of skeletal muscle fibres in newborn rats. *Journal of Neurocytology*, **5**, 591–604.

Kuffler, D.P., Thompson, W. & Jansen, J.K.S. (1980). The fate of foreign endplates in cross-innervated rat soleus muscle. *Proceedings of the Royal Society of London, Series B*, **208**, 189–222.

Lømo, T. & Slater, C.R. (1980). Acetylcholine sensitivity of developing ectopic nerve-muscle junctions in adult rat soleus muscles. *Journal of Physiology*, **303**, 173–89.

O'Brien, R.A.D., Ostberg, A.J.C. & Vrbova, G. (1978). Observations on the elimination of polyneuronal innervation in developing mammalian skeletal muscle. *Journal of Physiology*, **282**, 571–82.

O'Brien, R.A.D., Ostberg, A.J.C. & Vrbova, G. (1980). The effect of acetylcholine on the function and structure of the developing mammalian neuromuscular junction. *Neuroscience*, **5**, 1367–79.

Purves, D. & Lichtman, J.W. (1980). Elimination of synapses in the developing nervous system. *Science*, **210**, 153–7.

Redfern, P.A. (1970). Neuromuscular transmission in newborn rats. *Journal of Physiology*, **209**, 701–9.

Riley, D.A. (1976). Multiple axon branches innervating single endplates of kitten soleus myofibres. *Brain Research*, **110**, 158–61.

Riley, D.A. (1977). Spontaneous elimination of nerve terminals from the endplates of developing skeletal myofibres. *Brain Research*, **134**, 279–85.

Riley, D.A. (1981). Ultrastructural evidence for axon retraction during the spontaneous elimination of polyneuronal innervation of the rat soleus muscle. *Journal of Neurocytology*, **10**, 425–40.

Rosenthal, J.L. & Taraskevich, S.P. (1977). Reduction in multiaxonal innervation of the neuromuscular junction of the rat during development. *Journal of Physiology*, **270**, 299–310.

Thompson, W. & Jansen, J.K.S. (1977). The extent of sprouting of remaining motor units in partly denervated immature and adult rat soleus muscle. *Neuroscience*, **2**, 523–35.

Toutant, M., Bourgeois, J.P., Toutant, J.P., Renaud, D., Le Douarin, G. & Changeux, J.P. (1980). Chronic stimulation of the spinal cord in developing chick embryo causes the differentiation of multiple clusters of acetylcholine receptors in the posterior latissimus dorsi muscle. *Developmental Biology*, **76**, 384–95.

Excess presynaptic inputs in ganglia and the cerebellum

Crepel, F. (1982). Regression of functional synapses in the immature mammalian cerebellum. *Trends in Neurosciences*, **5**, 266–70.

Crepel, F., Mariani, J. & Delhaye-Bouchaud, N. (1976). Evidence for a multiple innervation of Purkinje cells by climbing fibres in the immature rat cerebellum. *Journal of Neurobiology*, **7**, 567–78.

Hume, R.I. & Purves, D. (1981). Geometry of neonatal neurones and the regulation of synapse elimination. *Nature, London*, **293**, 469–71.

Lichtman, J.W. (1977). The organisation of synaptic connections in the rat submandibular ganglion during post-natal development. *Journal of Physiology*, **273**, 155–78.

Lichtman, J.W. & Purves, D. (1980). The elimination of redundant preganglionic innervation to hamster sympathetic ganglion cells in early postnatal life. *Journal of Physiology*, **301**, 213–28.

Diffuse connections in the central nervous system

Fawcett, J.W. & Willshaw, D.J. (1982). Compound eyes project stripes on the optic tectum in *Xenopus*. *Nature, London*, **296**, 350–2.

Freeman, J.A. (1977). Possible regulatory function of acetylcholine receptor in maintenance of retinotectal synapses. *Nature, London*, **269**, 218–22.

Hubel, D.H., Wiesel, T.N. & Le Vay, S. (1977). Plasticity of ocular dominance columns in monkey striate cortex. *Philosophical Transactions of the Royal Society of London, Series B*, **278**, 377–404.

Innocenti, G.M. (1981). Growth and reshaping of axons in the establishment of visual callosal connections. *Science*, **212**, 824–7.

Keating, M.J. (1974). The role of visual function in the patterning of binocular visual connections. *British Medical Bulletin*, **30**, 145–51.

Law, M.I. & Constantine-Paton, M. (1981). Anatomy and physiology of experimentally induced striped tecta. *Journal of Neuroscience*, **1**, 741–59.

Levine, R.L. & Jacobson, M. (1975). Discontinuous mapping of retina onto tectum innervated by both eyes. *Brain Research*, **98**, 172–6.

Lund, R.D., Mitchell, D.E. & Henry, G.H. (1978). Squint-induced modification of callosal connections in cats. *Brain Research*, **144**, 169–72.

Meyer, R.L. (1982). Tetrodotoxin blocks the formation of ocular dominance columns in goldfish. *Science*, **218**, 589–91.

O'Leary, D.D.M., Stanfield, B.B. & Cowan, W.M. (1981). Evidence that the early postnatal restriction of the cells of origin of the callosal projection is due to the elimination of axon collaterals rather than to the death of neurons. *Developmental Brain Research*, **1**, 607–17.

Rakic, P. (1977). Prenatal development of the visual system in Rhesus monkey. *Philosophical Transactions of the Royal Society of London, Series B*, **278**, 245–60.

Rakic, P. (1981). Development of visual centres in the primate brain depends on binocular competition before birth. *Science*, **214**, 928–31.

Stanfield, B.B., O'Leary, D.D.M. & Fricks, C. (1982). Selective collateral elimination in early postnatal development restricts cortical distribution of rat pyramidal tract neurones. *Nature, London*, **298**, 371–3.

Swindale, N.V. (1981). Absence of ocular dominance patches in dark-reared cats. *Nature, London*, **290**, 332–3.

Wiesel, T.N. (1982). Postnatal development of the visual cortex and the influence of the environment. *Nature, London*, **299**, 583–91.

Modification of receptive fields in the visual cortex

Blakemore, C. & Mitchell, D.E. (1973). Environmental modification of the visual cortex and the neural basis of learning and memory. *Nature, London*, **241**, 467–8.

Blasdel, G. & Pettigrew, J.D. (1979). Degree of interocular synchrony required for maintenance of binocularity in kitten's visual cortex. *Journal of Neurophysiology*, **42**, 1692–710.

Cynader, M. & Mitchell, D.E. (1980). Prolonged sensitivity to monocular deprivation in dark-reared cats. *Journal of Neurophysiology*, **43**, 1026–40.

Duffy, F.H., Snodgrass, S.R., Burchfiel, J.L. & Conway, J.L. (1976). Bicuculline reversal of deprivation amblyopia in the cat. *Nature, London*, **260**, 256–7.

Hubel, D.H. (1982). Exploration of the primary visual cortex, 1955–1978. *Nature, London*, **299**, 515–24.

Hubel, D.H. & Wiesel, T.N. (1963). Receptive fields in striate cortex of very young, visually inexperienced kittens. *Journal of Neurophysiology*, **26**, 994–1002.

Hubel, D.H. & Wiesel, T.N. (1965). Binocular interaction in striate cortex of kittens reared with artificial squint. *Journal of Neurophysiology*, **28**, 1041–59.

Hubel, D.H. & Wiesel, T.N. (1970). The period of susceptibility to the physiological effects of unilateral eye closure in kittens. *Journal of Physiology*, **206**, 419–36.

Hubel, D.H. & Wiesel, T.N. (1979). Brain mechanisms of vision. *Scientific American*, **241** (Sept.), 130–45.

Kasamatsu, T., Pettigrew, J.D. & Ary, M. (1979). Restoration of visual cortical plasticity by local microperfusion of norepinephrine. *Journal of Comparative Neurology*, **185**, 163–82.

Kratz, K.E., Spear, P.D. & Smith, D.C. (1976). Postcritical-period reversal of effects of monocular deprivation in striate cortex cells in the cat. *Journal of Neurophysiology*, **39**, 501–11.

Lund, J.S., Boothe, R.G. & Lund, R.D. (1977). Development of neurons in the visual cortex (area 17) of the monkey (*Macaca nemestrina*): a Golgi study from fetal day 127 to postnatal maturity. *Journal of Comparative Neurology*, **176**, 149–88.

Martin, K.A.C., Ramachandran, V.S., Rao, V.M. & Whitteridge, D. (1979). Changes in ocular dominance induced in monocularly deprived lambs by stimulation with rotating gratings. *Nature, London*, **277**, 391–3.

O'Kusky, J. & Colonnier, M. (1982). Postnatal changes in the number of neurons and synapses in the visual cortex (area 17) of the macaque monkey: a stereological analysis in normal and monocularly deprived animals. *Journal of Comparative Neurology*, **210**, 291–306.

Pettigrew, J.D. (1974). The effect of visual experience on the development of stimulus specificity by kitten cortical neurons. *Journal of Physiology*, **237**, 49–74.

Pettigrew, J.D. (1978). The paradox of the critical period for striate cortex. In *Neuronal Plasticity*, ed. C.W. Cotman, pp. 311–30. New York: Raven Press.

Pettigrew, J., Olson, C. & Barlow, H.B. (1973). Kitten visual cortex: short-term, stimulus-induced changes in connectivity. *Science*, **180**, 1202–3.

Rauschecker, J.P. & Singer, W. (1981). The effects of early visual experience on the cat's visual cortex and their possible explanation by Hebb synapses. *Journal of Physiology*, **310**, 215–39.

Sillito, A.M. (1975). The contribution of inhibitory mechanisms to the receptive field properties of neurons in the striate cortex of the cat. *Journal of Physiology*, **250**, 305–29.

Stent, G.S. (1973). A physiological basis for Hebb's postulate of learning. *Proceedings of the National Academy of Sciences, USA*, **70**, 997–1001.

Wiesel, T.N. & Hubel, D.H. (1974). Ordered arrangement of orientation columns in monkeys lacking visual experience. *Journal of Comparative Neurology*, **158**, 307–18.

Synaptic reorganisation in other systems

Banks, M.S., Aslin, R.N. & Letson, R.D. (1975). Sensitive period for the development of human binocular vision. *Science*, **190**, 675–7.

Cooper, K.E., Ferguson, A.V. & Veale, W.L. (1980). Modification of thermoregulatory responses in rabbits reared at elevated environmental temperatures. *Journal of Physiology*, **303**, 165–72.

Dawson, N.J., Hellon, R.F., Herington, J.G. & Young, A.A. (1982). Facial thermal input in the caudal trigeminal nucleus of rats reared at 30 °C. *Journal of Physiology*, **333**, 545–54.

Knudsen, E.I., Knudsen, P.F. & Esterly, S.D. (1982). Early auditory experience modifies sound localisation in barn owls. *Nature, London*, **295**, 238–40.

Nottebohm, F. (1970). Ontogeny of bird song. *Science*, **167**, 950–6.

Van der Loos, H. & Woolsey, T.A. (1973). Somatosensory cortex: structural alterations following early injury to sense organs. *Science*, **179**, 395–8.

IV.3
Neural plasticity in normal adult animals

A plastic substance is pliable and will retain modifications in its shape. The nervous system is said to exhibit plasticity in that it undergoes changes following experience that result in learning and memory. Plasticity in axonal connections or synaptic effectiveness in response to experience-related activity is thought to be the basis of learning and memory, so there is an obvious interest in identifying and analysing any neuronal pathways that exhibit plasticity for clues to the mechanisms of learning. This chapter will deal with five examples of plasticity in the adult where some progress towards understanding the phenomenon is being made: modification of a reflex in the mollusc *Aplysia*, motor learning in the cerebellum, adaptation of the vestibulo-ocular reflex, long-term potentiation in the hippocampus, and classical conditioning in the red nucleus.

In the first three of these examples a stable behavioural change is induced in the animal, the site of the change is then identified, and finally the nature of the change and the synaptic mechanisms underlying it are analysed. Understanding of the learning that occurs in a simple reflex in *Aplysia* has reached as far as a detailed knowledge of biophysical changes in synaptic mechanisms. In the cerebellum the probable site of synaptic changes has been identified. The site and nature of adaptations which occur in the vestibulo-ocular reflex are still uncertain.

In the studies of the hippocampus and the red nucleus, neuronal connections are modified by activity delivered through stimulating electrodes. This approach offers the advantage that the site of modification is more easily identified and possibly more easily studied, but it then remains to be demonstrated how such modification has relevance to learning in the normal animal.

Modification of a reflex in *Aplysia*

Invertebrates display stable, adaptive changes in their behaviours, and their nervous systems have far fewer nerve cells than vertebrates, so they are an obvious starting point for investigating the neuronal basis of learning. The withdrawal reflex of the marine mollusc *Aplysia californica* (the sea hare) is a behaviour that exhibits stable long-term changes and it has been chosen by Kandel and his collaborators for analysis at the single-cell level (for a review see Kandel & Schwartz, 1982). The reflex consists of a brief defensive withdrawal of gills and siphon evoked by light tactile or electrical stimulation of the siphon. Repeated stimulation of the siphon causes a reduction of the withdrawal response that can last for up to several weeks. This is the phenomenon of *habituation*, the simplest form of learning. Strong electrical shocks to the head, which produce massive withdrawal responses, cause an immediate and long-lasting enhancement, or *sensitisation*, of the gill withdrawal reflex. A shock to the tail can also cause some sensitisation of the reflex, but more importantly, if a touch to the siphon is paired with the tail shock about 15 times, then there is a marked additional enhancement of the reflex which lasts for several weeks (Carew, Walters & Kandel, 1981). This shows that *classical conditioning* or *associative learning* of the withdrawal response has occurred, with the marked response to tail shock (the unconditioned stimulus) becoming associated with the siphon touch alone (the conditioned stimulus).

Much of the neuronal circuitry associated with the gill withdrawal reflex has been determined and the basis of sensitisation has now been largely established (fig. IV.9). The withdrawal reflex can be attributed to activity in a direct (monosynaptic) pathway from sensory neurons of the siphon mechanoreceptors to motor neurons of the gill and siphon musculature.

Fig. IV.9. Pathways for sensitisation of gill withdrawal reflex in *Aplysia*.

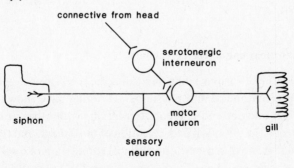

Enhancement of the withdrawal response is found to be caused by increased release of transmitter from the terminals of the sensory neurons. Activity in axons in the connectives running from the head region to the abdominal ganglion is thought to bring about this increase in release by a mechanism of *presynaptic facilitation* mediated by serotonin released from interneurons onto the sensory nerve's synapses on motor neurons. The evidence for this is as follows: serotonin applied to the sensory neurons produces a similar enhancement of transmission (Castellucci & Kandel, 1976; Brunelli, Castellucci & Kandel, 1976); a group of interneurons in the ganglion activated by head connectives (the L29 cells) produces a long-lasting facilitation of transmitter release if they are stimulated (Hawkins, Castellucci & Kandel, 1981), and these cells have all the morphological properties of serotonergic neurons; finally, contacts between these neurons, labelled with [^{3}H]serotonin, and sensory neurons labelled with horseradish peroxidase, were demonstrated by autoradiographic electron microscopy of the ganglion neuropile (Bailey *et al.*, 1981). Serotonin produces its effects on the sensory neuron terminals by increasing their intracellular concentration of cyclic AMP. This causes a reduction in the effective number of potassium channels in the membrane, which in turn allows a greater influx of calcium ions during depolarisations and hence a greater release of transmitter (Kandel & Schwartz, 1982).

The neuronal basis of the classical conditioning of the withdrawal reflex is currently under investigation. It is now apparent that presynaptic facilitation arising from the tail shock (the unconditioned stimulus) will be selectively enhanced in the terminals of the sensory neurons that are activated at the same time by siphon touch (the conditioned stimulus) (Hawkins *et al.*, 1982).

The depression of transmission accompanying habituation is due to a fall in the number of calcium channels in the presynaptic terminal, which is possibly caused by the rise in intracellular calcium ion concentration in the terminals following repeated activation of the pathway (Klein, Shapiro & Kandel, 1980).

Motor learning in the cerebellum

Evidence of various kinds implicates the cerebellum in the control of movement. Anatomical and physiological studies have shown that the cerebellum has afferent and efferent connections with other brain structures involved in the initiation and execution of movement, and that it also receives a wide range of sensory inputs. Focal stimulation of discrete areas of cerebellar cortex produces specific movements, and cerebellar lesions produce marked defects in movement co-ordination (ataxia). A closer analysis of the effects of cerebellar lesions shows that they produce defects in the retention and acquisition of learned movements. In cats, for example, eyelid blinking elicited by a puff of air directed at one eye can be conditioned to occur in response to an acoustic stimulus, and ablation of the ipsilateral cerebellar hemisphere selectively abolishes the conditioned responses without affecting the blinking reflex; moreover the conditioned response cannot be acquired following hemicerebellectomy (Lincoln, McCormick & Thompson, 1982).

When the details of circuitry in the cerebellar cortex were worked out by J.C. Eccles and others (see fig. IV.10), there was much speculation about how motor learning might be achieved in the cerebellum. The models proposed are all very similar (Marr, 1969; Albus, 1971; Gilbert, 1974). It is assumed that activity in Purkinje cells produces specific, 'elemental' movements. Each Purkinje cell receives a strong input from a single climbing fibre, which may be closely connected with the sensory receptors for the movement associated with that Purkinje cell, or with the cortical area where the movement is initiated. The Purkinje cells also receive weaker inputs from a wide range of sensory receptors via the parallel fibres of the granule cells, which are connected to the mossy fibre inputs to the cerebellum. Activity in the climbing fibre was envisaged by Marr as somehow increasing the efficacy of any parallel fibre–Purkinje cell synapses that were also active at the same time (fig. IV.10). In the above example of

Fig. IV.10. Motor learning in cerebellar cortex. Synchronous activity in a climbing fibre and a parallel fibre is thought to modify the strength of the synapse of the parallel fibre on the Purkinje cell dendrite.

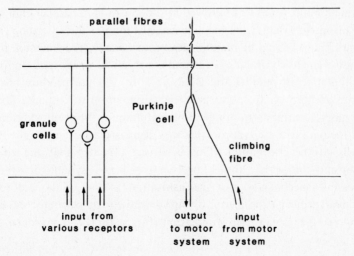

conditioned eyelid blinking, the puff of air would produce activity in the climbing fibres that synapse on Purkinje cells associated with eyelid movement, the acoustic stimulus would produce activity in parallel fibres, and transmission at the synapses of the parallel fibres on the eyelid Purkinje cells would be stably enhanced because of the synchrony between parallel fibres and climbing fibres. Conditioning would be achieved when the acoustic stimulus alone could excite the Purkinje cells via the parallel fibres and thereby elicit the blink.

Albus (1971) produced a similar theory, but reasoned that the system would be more efficient and inherently more stable if transmission at the parallel fibre–Purkinje cell synapses was made *less* effective by conjoint activity in the climbing fibres. Experiments are now being performed to test the interaction between the climbing and parallel fibres on the Purkinje cells, and the results are supporting the Albus theory (Andersen, 1982). In a study on conscious monkeys that were learning a hand movement parallel-fibre-induced activity was assayed in Purkinje cells as simple spikes, and climbing-fibre-induced activity was assayed in the same cells as complex spikes (the climbing fibre input is more powerful than the parallel fibre input). In the area of the cerebellum associated with arm movements Purkinje cells were found in which there were transient increases in complex spike activity during the learning period, and in these cells there was a decrease in simple spike activity that persisted after the complex spike activity had returned to normal (Gilbert & Thach, 1977).

In an elegant study by Ito and his coworkers parallel fibres in the vestibular cerebellum were stimulated via the ipsilateral vestibular nerve, climbing fibres were stimulated where they originate in the inferior olive, and activity was recorded in Purkinje cells. Conjoint stimulation of parallel and climbing fibres was followed by a depression in parallel fibre synaptic transmission that lasted in some cases as long as the recording from the Purkinje cell could be maintained (up to 1 hour). Transmission from the unstimulated contralateral vestibular nerve was unaffected, and random stimulation of parallel and climbing fibres did not produce changes in parallel fibre synaptic transmission. Stimulation of climbing fibres and conjoint iontophoretic application of glutamate, the presumed transmitter at the parallel fibre synapses, led to a decreased sensitivity of the Purkinje cells to the transmitter. This is strong evidence that the change in transmission of the parallel fibre synapses is post-synaptic in origin. One possible mechanism is a desensitisation of any glutamate receptors activated during the period of high intradentritic calcium concentration following climbing fibre stimulation (Ito, Sakurai & Tongroach, 1982).

Adaptation of the vestibulo-ocular reflex

Evolution has endowed vertebrates with several eye movement reflexes which improve visual performance by eliminating image movements on the retina. Two of these reflexes utilise negative feedback of retinal image velocity to offset the retinal image movement: the optokinetic reflex, common to all vertebrates, responds to movement of images across the whole retina and appears to be useful when an animal makes translational movements relative to its environment; in higher vertebrates there is also a pursuit reflex which is tuned to small moving images in the foveal region and which allows the animal to 'track' moving objects. The requirement for visual information to activate them makes both these reflexes relatively slow, with delays in onset of approximately 100 milliseconds. In contrast, the vestibulo-ocular reflex (VOR), which offsets rotations of the head with equal and opposite smooth rotations of the eye, does not use visual feedback and is much faster. Head rotations are sensed in the semicircular canals and fed directly via the brain stem to the extraocular muscles (fig. IV.11). In order to compensate for fast head turns the VOR has a very short latency. There is a total delay of only about 10 milliseconds between activation of the semicircular canals and onset of compensatory eye rotation, and this is achieved by having only two or three synapses in the VOR pathway.

The ability of the VOR to function without visual feedback led to the belief that its gain of approximately unity (eye angular velocity divided by head angular velocity) was fixed. However, it is now clear that the VOR has to be adaptable throughout life, since any changes in vestibular sensitivity, central transmission or eye mechanics associated with growth and aging

Fig. IV.11. Pathways of the reflexes stabilising retinal images.

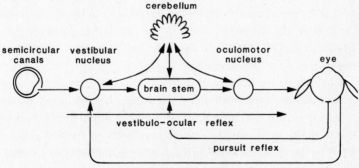

have to be accommodated if efficient vision is to be preserved. Recent experimentation with various optical devices in animals ranging from fish to man has indeed revealed that the gain of the VOR is not fixed but can adapt to reduce or eliminate any retinal image-slip associated with head turns. In monkeys, for example, constant wearing of two-fold magnifying spectacles produces after 1 week a nearly two-fold gain increase in the VOR, and reducing spectacles produce correspondingly reduced VOR gains (Miles & Eighmy, 1980). These adaptations persist until the spectacles are removed, whereupon the VOR gradually reverts to normal. The VOR therefore seems to be a relatively simple system for studying adult neuronal plasticity.

Investigation of the VOR has centred on identifying the source of the error signal which brings about the gain change and the site of the gain change itself. When an animal with an inappropriately adapted VOR turns its head, images will slip across its retina. Retinal image-slip signals, which are available in the brain to control the tracking reflexes, must therefore be the ultimate source of the error signal. The pursuit reflex has to be used in such animals to keep a stationary object on the fovea during head turns, so the output of the pursuit reflex could also provide an error signal. Whatever its source, the error signal must then cause gradual gain changes in the VOR pathway by combining somehow with concomitant vestibular activity. The obvious place for this to occur is the cerebellum: retinal image-slip could appear on the climbing fibres and alter the strength of the synapses of parallel fibres carrying vestibular signals, and output from the Purkinje cells would then control the VOR by feeding into the motor pathway to the eye muscles (Ito, 1972). This would put the site of the gain change in the cerebellum, and consistent with this is the observation that cerebellar lesions in cats abolish not only VOR plasticity but also previously adapted gain changes (Robinson, 1976). However, in monkeys with an adapted VOR sudden changes in velocity of the head evoke adapted, compensatory changes in the velocity of the eyes long before any changes in the discharge rate can be detected in Purkinje cells (Miles, Braitman & Dow, 1980), so at least in this species the gain change is unlikely to be in the cerebellum.

Changes in the activity in the vestibular primary afferents or in first-order neurons in the vestibular nucleus have been detected in cats wearing reversing prisms (Keller & Precht, 1979) but not in monkeys (Lisberger & miles, 1980), so in cats the change may occur in the first elements of the VOR pathway. Following VOR adaptation in monkeys, changes occur in the optokinetic reflex but not the pursuit reflex, suggesting that the modified element is between the stages where these reflexes enter the VOR pathway. It would appear, therefore, that in the monkey the modifications occur in the brain stem (Miles & Lisberger, 1981). At present there is no indication of the precise location in the brain stem and hence the cellular nature of the change is unknown.

Long-term potentiation in the hippocampus

The hippocampus is the phylogenetically older part of the cerebral cortex connected with the limbic system. There is considerable evidence that it is important in acquiring and retaining some forms of memory. Damage to the hippocampus is known to produce deficits in memory in humans. Rats also lose the memory of how best to use a maze to get a food reward, and cannot relearn following hippocampal lesions (Olton, Walker & Gage, 1978). Moreover a high proportion of the neurons in the hippocampus in conscious rats show alterations in their firing patterns that are specific to the animal's position in a familiar environment (O'Keefe & Dostrovsky, 1971; O'Keefe, 1976).

Synaptic transmission in the hippocampus was first studied in anaesthetised rabbits by directly stimulating one of the main afferent tracts, the perforant path (Bliss & Lømo, 1973) (fig. IV.12). The perforant path arises in the entorhinal cortex and terminates on dendrites of the granule cells of the dentate area of the hippocampus. The excitatory post-synaptic potential evoked in the granule cells by perforant path stimulation can be recorded with an extracellular electrode as a synaptic wave caused by the flow of current into the dendrites. With sufficient stimulation there can also be a superimposed spike caused by the synchronous firing of an action potential in some granule cells. Single stimuli to the perforant path every

Fig. IV.12. Long-term potentiation of evoked responses in dendritic layer of dentate area of hippocampus following stimulation of the perforant path. Dashed and continuous lines in trace, before and after long-term potentiation respectively; epsp, excitatory post-synaptic potential. (After Bliss & Lømo, 1973.)

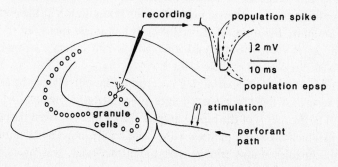

few seconds produce a constant post-synaptic activation of the granule cells, but if an extra train of stimuli at a frequency of 10–100 hertz is applied for 10 or more seconds, substantial short- and long-term changes in transmission occur. During the train there is a potentiation of transmission, as evidenced by increases in wave and spike amplitude and a decrease in spike latency. Immediately after the train there is a period of depression lasting for up to a minute, but thereafter there is a return of potentiation which can last for hours in anaesthetised animals and for over a week in conscious animals. This latter phenomenon has been called long-term potentiation (LTP), and it has been observed in several other pathways within the hippocampus. Elsewhere in the nervous system potentiation can be produced by trains of stimuli, but in all cases high frequencies and long trains are required to produce the effect and the potentiation lasts only for minutes or at most hours.

LTP does not occur unless a sufficient number of axons are activated by the conditioning train of stimuli. This implies that there is some kind of co-operative interaction between axons on the post-synaptic cells. However, where two separate pathways that can both be potentiated converge on the same cells, LTP of one pathway causes only a short-term depression in the other and does not affect its potentiation, and this applies even where both pathways converge on the same general region of the dendrites (Dunwiddie & Lynch, 1978). It is not known whether there are co-operative or competitive interactions between even more closely converging axons, for example between stimulated and unstimulated axons of the same pathway.

The subcellular site of the enhancement of transmission is not yet clear. Fifkova & Van Harreveld (1977) performed an electron microscopic analysis of the dentate area following perforant path stimulation and found a significant increase in dendrite spine diameters only in the region of perforant path termination. An increased conductance between the dendritic spine synapses and the dendritic shaft might accompany this structural change and this could be one possible post-synaptic mechanism for LTP. More recently it has been found that a perfusate of the dentate area contains more glutamate ions following potentiation of the perforant path (Dolphin, Errington & Bliss, 1982). If glutamate turns out to be the transmitter of the perforant path then this would indicate strongly that there is also a presynaptic basis for LTP.

Further progress on determining the mechanism of LTP may be possible with the use of the hippocampal slice preparation (Lynch & Schubert, 1980). The geometry of the hippocampus allows slices of fresh tissue to be taken in which the major pathways are functionally intact and exhibit LTP *in vitro*. The roles of ions, transmitters and intracellular messengers in LTP can be more easily assessed in these slices than in the intact animal. Some early results suggest that, as in *Aplysia*, modulation of presynaptic calcium currents and hence transmitter output occurs during LTP (Turner, Bambridge & Miller, 1982). However, more studies on the intact animal will be necessary if it is to be demonstrated that LTP occurs naturally in the hippocampus and that it is associated with learning.

Classical conditioning in the red nucleus

The red nucleus is a midbrain structure involved in motor control. It receives inputs from the cerebral cortex directly and from the cerebellum via the nucleus interpositus, and its axons project to the motor circuitry of the spinal cord. An indication that the red nucleus might be important in some motor learning situations was provided by experiments of Smith (1970), who was investigating classical conditioning of forelimb flexion in cats. Avoidance flexion, the response to a shock to the skin of the forelimb (the unconditioned stimulus), was paired with the sound of a tone until the tone itself (the conditioned stimulus) was able to evoke the response. Lesions to the red nucleus were then found to impair the ability of trained animals to respond to the tone, although they were still able to perform normal movements with the forelimb.

In other experiments strong electrical stimulation of the red nucleus evoked flexion and could serve as the unconditioned stimulus for conditioning the tone. It was also found that weak stimuli applied to the red nucleus below the threshold for movement could evoke strong flexions after they had been paired with forelimb shocks for several days. Tsukahara, Oda & Notsu (1981) have refined the latter experiment by applying the weak stimulation to the cortical pathway to the red nucleus, rather than to the red nucleus itself, and have achieved the same enhanced response to the stimulation (fig. IV.13). Several observations make it likely

Fig. IV.13. Classical conditioning in the red nucleus. CS, conditioned stimulus (initially ineffective in causing limb flexion); US, unconditioned stimulus. (After Tsukahara *et al.*, 1981.)

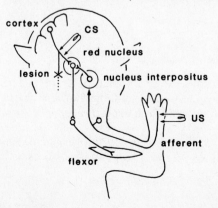

that the end result of this conditioning is a change only at the cortical input
to the red nucleus. First, the experiments were performed following lesions
to the corticofugal pathway that spared only the corticorubral tract.
Secondly, flexion produced by stimulation of the pathway to the red
nucleus from the nucleus interpositus was not enhanced following training.
Finally the minimal latency of the enhanced response is consistent with the
time taken for activity to reach the muscles via the corticorubrospinal tract.

Following training, the enhancement in performance in response to
various levels of corticorubral stimulation is modelled accurately by
assuming an enhancement of transmission in the corticorubral synapses,
whereas the performance predicted by an increase in excitability of red
nucleus neurons fits the observed data less well. Direct electrophysiological
investigation will be necessary to confirm whether it is indeed synaptic
transmission that is enhanced, and detailed structural studies should reveal
whether there is sprouting or other pre- or post-synaptic changes in the
synapses. The way in which limb shocks enhance corticorubral transmission is also of special interest. It probably involves an interaction between
activity in the corticorubral synapses and activity induced by the limb
shock in synapses from the nucleus interpositus.

Conclusion

The basis of the associative learning that has been demonstrated in
Aplysia, the cerebellum and the red nucleus is a modification of synaptic
effectiveness of those inputs that are active in synchrony with other inputs
on the same cell. Repeated use of a pathway appears to enhance
transmission in the hippocampus, but it is too early to say whether the
phenomenon of LTP is a manifestation of any learning mechanism that
occurs in the hippocampus. The significance of VOR plasticity to other
forms of learning also remains to be established.

References

Modification of a reflex in Aplysia

Bailey, C.H., Hawkins, R.D., Chen, M.C. & Kandel, E.R. (1981). Interneurons
involved in mediation and modulation of gill-withdrawal reflex in *Aplysia*. IV.
Morphological basis of pre-synaptic facilitation. *Journal of Neurophysiology*,
45, 340–60.

Brunelli, M., Castellucci, V. & Kandel, E.R. (1976). Synaptic facilitation and
behavioural sensitization in *Aplysia*: possible role of serotonin and cyclic AMP.
Science, **194**, 1178–81.

Carew, T.J., Walters, E.T. & Kandel, E.R. (1981). Classical conditioning in a simple withdrawal reflex in *Aplysia californica. Journal of Neuroscience*, **1**, 1426–37.

Castellucci, V. & Kandel, E.R. (1976). Pre-synaptic facilitation as a mechanism for behavioural sensitization in *Aplysia. Science*, **194**, 1176–8.

Hawkins, R.D., Abrams, T.W., Carew, T.J. & Kandel, E.R. (1982). A cellular mechanism of classical conditioning in *Aplysia*: activity-dependent amplification of presynaptic facilitation. *Science*, **219**, 400–5.

Hawkins, R.D., Castellucci, V.F. & Kandel, E.R. (1981). Interneurons involved in mediation and modulation of the gill-withdrawal reflex in *Aplysia*. II. Identified neurons produce heterosynaptic facilitation contributing to behavioural sensitization. *Journal of Neurophysiology*, **45**, 315–26.

Kandel, E.R. (1981). Calcium and the control of synaptic strength by learning. *Nature, London*, **293**, 697–700.

Kandel, E.R. & Schwartz, J.H. (1982). Molecular biology of an elementary form of learning: modulation of transmitter release through cyclic AMP-dependent protein kinase. *Science*, **218**, 433–43.

Klein, M., Shapiro, E. & Kandel, E.R. (1980). Synaptic plasticity and the modulation of the Ca^{++} current. *Journal of Experimental Biology*, **89**, 117–57.

Motor learning in the cerebellum

Albus, J.S. (1971). A theory of cerebellar function. *Mathematical Biosciences*, **10**, 25–61.

Andersen, P. (1982). Cerebellar synaptic plasticity – putting theories to the test. *Trends in Neurosciences*, **5**, 324–5.

Gilbert, P.F.C. (1974). A theory of memory that explains the function and structure of the cerebellum. *Brain Research*, **70**, 1–18.

Gilbert, P.F.C. & Thach, W.T. (1977). Purkinje cell activity during motor learning. *Brain Research*, **128**, 309–28.

Ito, M., Sakurai, M. & Tongroach, P. (1982). Climbing fibre induced depressions of both mossy fibre responsiveness and glutamate sensitivity of cerebellar Purkinje cells. *Journal of Physiology*, **324**, 113–34.

Lincoln, J.S., McCormick, D.A. & Thompson, R.F. (1982). Ipsilateral cerebellar lesions prevent learning of the classically conditioned nictitating membrane/eyelid response. *Brain Research*, **242**, 190–3.

Marr, D. (1969). A theory of cerebellar cortex. *Journal of Physiology*, **202**, 437–70.

Adaptation of the vestibulo-ocular reflex

Ito, M. (1972). Neural design of the cerebellar motor control system. *Brain Research*, **40**, 81–4.

Keller, E.L. & Precht, W. (1979). Adaptive modification of central vestibular neurons in response to visual stimulation through reversing prisms. *Journal of Neurophysiology*, **42**, 896–911.

Lisberger, S.G. & Miles, F.A. (1980). Role of primate medial vestibular nucleus in long-term adaptive plasticity of vestibulo-ocular reflex. *Journal of Neurophysiology*, **43**, 1725–45.

Miles, F.A., Braitman, D.J. & Dow, B.M. (1980). Long-term adaptive changes in primate vestibulo-ocular reflex. IV. Electrophysiological observations in flocculus of adapted monkeys. *Journal of Neurophysiology*, **43**, 1477–93.

Miles, F.A. & Eighmy, B.B. (1980). Long-term adaptive changes in primate vestibulo-ocular reflex. I. Behavioural observations. *Journal of Neurophysiology*, **43**, 1406–25.

Miles, F.A. & Lisberger, S.G. (1981). Plasticity of the vestibulo-ocular reflex: a new hypothesis. *Annual Review of Neurosciences*, **4**, 273–99.

Robinson, D.A. (1976). Adaptive gain control of vestibulo-ocular reflex by the cerebellum. *Journal of Neurophysiology*, **39**, 954–69.

Long-term potentiation in the hippocampus

Bliss, R.V.P. & Lømo, T. (1973). Long-lasting potentiation of synaptic transmission in the dentate area of the anaesthetised rabbit following stimulation of the perforant path. *Journal of Physiology*, **232**, 331–6.

Dolphin, A.C., Errington, M.L. & Bliss, R.V.P. (1982). Long-term potentiation of the perforant path *in vivo* is associated with increased glutamate release. *Nature, London*, **297**, 496–8.

Dunwiddie, T. & Lynch, G. (1978). Long-term potentiation and depression of synaptic responses in the rat hippocampus: localisation and frequency dependency. *Journal of Physiology*, **276**, 353–67.

Fifkova, E. & Van Harreveld, A. (1977). Long-lasting morphological changes in dendritic spines of dentate granular cells following stimulation of the entorhinal area. *Journal of Neurocytology*, **6**, 211–30.

Lynch, G. & Schubert, P. (1980). The use of *in vitro* brain slices for multidisciplinary studies of synaptic function. *Annual Review of Neuroscience*, **3**, 1–22.

O'Keefe, J. (1976). Place units in the hippocampus of the freely-moving rat. *Experimental Neurology*, **51**, 78–109.

O'Keefe, J. & Dostrovsky, J. (1971). The hippocampus as a spatial map. Preliminary evidence from unit activity in the freely-moving rat. *Brain Research*, **34**, 171–5.

Olton, D.S., Walker, J.A. & Gage, F.H. (1978). Hippocampal connections in spatial discrimination. *Brain Research*, **139**, 295–308.

Turner, R.W., Bambridge, K.G. & Miller, J.J. (1982). Calcium-induced long-term potentiation in the hippocampus. *Neuroscience*, **7**, 1411–16.

Classical conditioning in the red nucleus

Smith, A.M. (1970). The effects of rubral lesions and stimulation conditioned forelimb flexion responses in the cat. *Physiology and Behaviour*, **5**, 1121–6.

Tsukahara, M., Oda, Y. & Notsu, T. (1981). Classical conditioning mediated by the red nucleus in the cat. *Journal of Neuroscience*, **1**, 72–9.

IV.4

Nerve injury and trophic effects

Introduction

It is common knowledge that denervated limbs become wasted and that the healthy state of the limb tissues is restored only following successful reinnervation. Closer examination of denervated target cells shows that they undergo marked changes in many of their properties. It is apparent, therefore, that normal target cell properties are maintained in some way by the nerve. This influence of the nerve on its target is called the orthograde trophic effect.

Orthograde trophic effects could be mediated either by post-synaptic electrical activity evoked by the nerve or by substances synthesised in the nerve cell body, transported along the axons and released onto the target cells (fig. IV.14). The neurotransmitter itself could also have a direct trophic effect on post-synaptic cells quite apart from any trophic effect of the electrical activity it induces. In mammalian skeletal muscle the trophic

Fig. IV.14. Orthograde and retrograde trophic influences between neuron, glia and target cells.

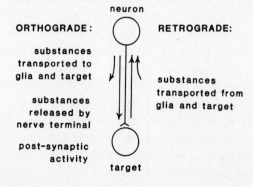

effect is found to be mediated predominantly by action potentials in the muscle fibres; substances released by the motor nerves have little or no effect on most muscle properties, as might be expected from the relatively small size and localised distribution of the nerve terminals in relation to the bulk of the muscle. However, properties of the synaptic region of the muscle fibres are probably influenced directly by neurotransmitter or other nerve-released substances, and other innervated tissues and glial cells appear to be maintained by trophic substances released by nerves.

Effects of axotomy are not restricted to cells distal to the site of injury. Neurons which have been disconnected from their targets also undergo characteristic morphological changes which have been termed 'chromatolysis', and there are accompanying changes in physiological and biochemical properties of the neurons, changes in the satellite cells, and changes in synaptic connections. There is considerable evidence that these changes are mediated at least partly by the interruption of the retrograde transport of a trophic factor, or 'retrophin', which is released by target tissues and probably also by glial cells, and which is taken up by the axons (fig. IV.14). Nerve Growth Factor appears to be a retrophin for sympathetic and sensory nerves, and evidence for the existence of retrophins which are effective on other neurons is beginning to accumulate.

Orthograde trophic effects on peripheral nerve

Evidence for the existence of a trophic effect maintaining the integrity of peripheral nerves is provided by observations on the earliest changes in the distal nerve stump after it has been separated from the cell body by axotomy. Failure in the spontaneous and evoked release of transmitter occurs first, accompanied and possibly caused by disruption of the nerve terminal by its associated glial cells. Failure is delayed if the nerve is transected further away from the muscle, and the signal for failure appears to travel distally from the site of nerve transection at a rate of about 1 centimetre per hour in mammals (Miledi & Slater, 1970). A similar signal may trigger the first visible structural change in the myelin – the fragmentation into ovoids – which also spreads distally at about the same rate (Lubinska, 1977). The changes are probably initiated by a drop in the level of a substance supplied by the cell body rather than by the entry of substances into the axon at the site of injury, since segments of nerve isolated by two transections degenerate more slowly (Lubinska, 1982). Loss of trophic substance probably initiates the subsequent phagocytosis of the axon by the Schwann cells, which also engulf their own myelin. Mitosis of the Schwann cells occurs too, but this may be triggered by a component of the breakdown products of the myelin membrane (Salzer & Bunge, 1980). The Schwann cells then gradually atrophy and eventually degenerate (Weinberg & Spencer, 1978).

The nature of the signal passing from axon to Schwann cell remains unclear. Labelled proteins transported down the axon from the cell body do not appear to cross into the Schwann cells, although some membrane components do (Droz, 1979). Physical transfer of material may not even be necessary if the trophic effect is mediated by contact between the Schwann cell and a component of the axon membrane.

Orthograde trophic effects on mammalian skeletal muscle

The major changes that have been identified in muscle cells following denervation are summarised in fig. IV.15. They include a small depolarisation of the resting potential, changes in contractile properties and junctional and extrajunctional membrane properties, and eventually atrophy of fibres. One other major change in muscle is of course the lack of action potentials, and it is now clear that the loss of activity is responsible for most of the changes in muscle properties following denervation. In the experiment which first showed this conclusively, extrajunctional acetylcholine sensitivity was assayed in muscles which were denervated but stimulated directly through electrodes implanted next to them. It was found that increases in sensitivity associated with denervation did not

Fig. IV.15. Changes in peripheral nerve and muscle which are caused directly or indirectly by loss of orthograde trophic influences following axotomy. ACh, acetylcholine.

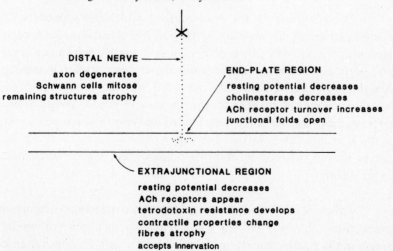

DISTAL NERVE ———▶

axon degenerates
Schwann cells mitose
remaining structures atrophy

END-PLATE REGION

resting potential decreases
cholinesterase decreases
ACh receptor turnover increases
junctional folds open

EXTRAJUNCTIONAL REGION

resting potential decreases
ACh receptors appear
tetrodotoxin resistance develops
contractile properties change
fibres atrophy
accepts innervation

occur in the stimulated muscles, whereas muscles with intact nerves in which activity had been blocked with small cuffs containing local anaesthetic developed changes characteristic of the denervated state (Lømo & Rosenthal, 1972). It has since been demonstrated that other extrajunctional membrane properties and junctional cholinesterase are also maintained by activity (e.g. Westgaard, 1975; Weinberg & Hall, 1979).

It has also been shown that the particular pattern of electrical activity delivered through electrodes either to denervated muscles (Lømo, West-gaard & Dahl, 1974) or to muscles with their nerves intact (Salmons & Sreter, 1976) can bring about changes in the contractile properties of the muscle that are as extensive as those described after nerves between slow and fast muscles were crossed (Buller, Eccles & Eccles, 1960). Thus continuous low-frequency activation (a pattern of firing characteristic of motor neurons innervating slow, oxidative motor units) slows the contrac-tion time of fast glycolytic muscles and causes them to develop more mitochondria and capillaries. On the other hand, the same number of impulses delivered in intermittent high-frequency bursts (a pattern charac-teristic of fast, fatiguable motor units) converts slow muscles into fast muscles. This control of muscle type by pattern of muscle use is an eminently sensible, adaptive strategy.

It is therefore clear that action potentials in mammalian skeletal muscle play a major part in the trophic maintenance of its properties. Is there also an additional trophic effect independent of muscle activity, mediated directly by acetylcholine or by other substances that may be released by motor nerve terminals (e.g. Chan-Palay *et al.*, 1982)? Several different experimental approaches have been taken to try to answer this question:

Effects of blockade of axonal transport. Colchicine applied locally to peripheral nerves inhibits axonal transport and eventually causes nerve degeneration, presumably through depletion of trophic substances in the distal portion of the nerve. Denervation-like changes develop in muscles when their nerves are treated with colchicine, and this occurs before the nerves degenerate and cease to activate the muscle. It was thought at first that these changes could be attributed to reduced release of a trophic agent, but this is made unlikely by the observation that colchicine causes similar changes directly when it reaches the muscle fibres via the circulation (Lømo, 1974).

Effects of blockade of activity. If nerve conduction or synaptic transmission is blocked and the nerve remains intact, denervation-like changes in the inactive muscle are found to be less well developed than in fully denervated muscles. However, it cannot be concluded that intact but inactive nerves have a residual trophic effect on muscle properties, because the presence of the degenerating nerve in the denervated muscle produces directly, and in an as yet unknown way, extra denervation-like changes (e.g. Cangiano & Lutzemberger, 1980). Attempts have been made to prolong blockade to allow the effects of nerve degeneration to subside, but where differences between blocked and denervated muscles persist it cannot be guaranteed that all nerve-evoked activity has been prevented. Complete blockade with botulinum toxin produced convergence of properties in blocked and denervated muscles (Brown, Hopkins & Keynes, 1982), but the toxin may itself prevent release of any putative trophic factor. These experiments therefore remain inconclusive.

Effects of nerve-derived substances on muscles in organ culture. Cultures of embryonic muscles provide a convenient system for analysing nerve-derived substances which might promote synaptogenesis (chapter III.3). In a similar way organ cultures of adult muscles have been used to determine whether such substances can inhibit or reverse denervation-induced changes. An extract of various tissues, including nerve, can stimulate the synthesis of cholinesterase at the end-plate of organ-cultured muscles (Davey, Younkin & Younkin, 1979), and an extract of spinal cord can alter properties of the action potential and acetylcholine receptors of denervated muscles towards those of the innervated state (Kuromi, Gonoi & Hosegawa, 1979). It remains to be seen whether the agent or agents responsible are active at normal motor nerve terminals.

Short-term organ cultures of muscles have also been used to investigate the fall in resting potential that occurs following denervation. The time of onset of the fall shows a dependence on nerve stump length that suggests it could be under the control of a trophic substance (Albuquerque, Schuh & Kauffman, 1971). If the freshly denervated muscle is incubated *in vitro*, the fall is delayed by cholinergic agonists and advanced by antagonists, indicating that acetylcholine itself might be acting as the trophic agent (Bray, Forrest & Hubbard, 1982). Oddly, however, the drop can occur in the presence of miniature end-plate potentials, i.e. with an intact nerve terminal present on the muscle fibre. It has therefore been postulated that the trophic effect is exerted at least partly by non-quantally released acetylcholine, which might stop before the terminal degenerates. The effect of acetylcholine is to some extent mimicked by exposing the muscles to a calcium ionophore, suggesting that the transmitter mediates its effects via the calcium ions that enter the muscle cell through the ion channels in the post-junctional membrane (Forrest *et al.*, 1981). It is possible that transmitter-mediated calcium entry might not only maintain other properties of the junctional region, but also play an important role in synaptogenesis. Calcium ions might in addition mediate the trophic effects of action potentials in muscle.

Orthograde trophic effects in other tissues

Neurons. In experiments performed earlier this century assays of end-organ responses to intravenous infusions of neurotransmitters demonstrated that denervated (i.e. decentralised) sympathetic ganglia developed supersensitivity to acetylcholine following denervation. Similar changes in denervated parasympathetic ganglion cells in the heart have been detected by recording intracellular responses to iontophoretically applied acetylcholine (Kuffler, Dennis & Harris, 1971). If the preganglionic nerve is allowed to regenerate into the cardiac ganglion this sensitivity is reduced in many ganglion cells before activity can be evoked in them by nerve stimulation, suggesting that a trophic agent independent of post-synaptic activity is responsible for maintaining the normal sensitivity (Dennis & Sargent, 1979).

The relative contributions of post-synaptic activity and trophic substances to maintenance of sympathetic ganglion sensitivity have not been investigated, but the regulation of the enzyme tyrosine hydroxylase in the superior cervical ganglion has received considerable attention. Decentralisation of the ganglion in the adult produces a gradual decline in the level of tyrosine hydroxylase (Hendry, Iversen & Black, 1973), suggesting that it is under trophic control by the preganglionic nerves. Activity in the *presynaptic* terminals appears to have the important regulatory influence, because a brief period of intense preganglionic stimulation produces a significant increase in tyrosine hydroxylase in the ganglion 3 days later, whereas the same stimulation applied to the ganglion cells via the post-synaptic nerve is ineffective (Chalazonitis & Zigmond, 1980). Thus presynaptic activity probably increases the release of a trophic agent from the nerve terminals. The effect of presynaptic stimulation is antagonised by the ganglion-blocking drug hexamethonium, suggesting that the trophic agent could be the transmitter itself (Chalazonitis & Zigmond, 1980).

The transmitter noradrenaline in the post-ganglionic nerves also appears to be the trophic agent responsible for maintenance of the pineal gland. Denervation of the pineal, or simply a period of relative inactivity, produces supersensitivity to noradrenaline, whereas presynaptic activity reduces the sensitivity and increases synthesis of the enzyme which produces melatonin in the gland. Noradrenaline probably mediates these effects by hyperpolarising the gland cells (see review by Zigmond & Bowers, 1981).

In the CNS denervation (deafferentation) can lead to cell shrinkage and even death of the post-synaptic neurons. For example, cells in the lateral geniculate nucleus degenerate when the optic nerve is cut (Matthews, Cowan & Powell, 1960). Activity is at least partly responsible for maintaining these cells because artificial closure of one eye leads to cell shrinkage (Wiesel & Hubel, 1963).

Frog slow muscle. Some muscles in the frog do not normally have an action potential, but instead are depolarised entirely by acetylcholine released from terminals distributed along the fibres. An action potential mechanism does develop on denervated fibres, and it is suppressed when the nerve regenerates (Schmidt & Stefani, 1977). Paralysis with α-bungarotoxin also induces the action potential mechanism, which indicates that acetylcholine is likely to be the agent which maintains the normal non-excitable state of the muscle (Miledi & Uchitel, 1981).

Sensory end-organs. Sensory neurons also exert trophic effects on their end-organs. Taste buds, for example, atrophy rapidly following section of the gustatory nerves and return to normal following reinnervation. The maintenance is to some extent non-specific, in that non-gustatory sensory nerves will reinstate the structure of the end-organ, whereas motor nerves will not (Zalewski, 1969). However, little more is known about the nature of this trophic support. It is possible that the substances released by the nerve at its central terminals are also released in the periphery and maintain the end-organ.

Invertebrate nerve and muscle. Invertebrate nerves are supported trophically by the cell body, because the peripheral stump of a severed nerve degenerates. However, in some cases the degeneration is very slow (action potentials can be conducted for several months) and the severed ends can fuse together again (Hoy, Bittner & Kennedy, 1967). Crustacean leg muscles atrophy following denervation but do not develop supersensitivity to the excitatory transmitter glutamate (Frank, 1974). A small increase in sensitivity can be detected in denervated insect leg muscles (Usherwood, 1969). The nature of these trophic effects has received scant attention. Activity is important for transforming a particular fast muscle into a slow muscle in lobsters during development (Govind & Kent, 1982), and it is probably also important for maintaining muscle properties in the adult.

Effects of nerves on limb regeneration. One well-known trophic action of nerves is their ability to support the regrowth of amputated limbs in Urodela and Crustacea. It seems that this action is non-specific, depending on quantity rather than type of nerves (see review by Singer, 1974). The regrowth of the amputated limb is due to mitosis of mesenchymal cells at the stump tip, and it is possible that the action of the nerves is mediated by the same or similar agents that induce glial and fibroblast mitosis during development of peripheral nerves (see section on neuron–glia relationships, p. 53).

Nerve injury and retrograde trophic effects

The most obvious structural change in neurons which have been disconnected from their periphery is dispersion of the aggregates of ribosomes and endoplasmic reticulum in the cell body. This was first observed last century in the light microscope as a dissolution of the Nissl substance, and the term chromatolysis was coined to describe it. Other structural changes were detected with the light microscope, and a proportion of cells were also seen to die. A wide variety of techniques have since been used to analyse the chromatolytic changes that occur in and around axotomised neurons. These changes are summarised in fig. IV.16. Biophysical and biochemical investigations have revealed transient increases in RNA and protein synthesis and turnover rates not only in the nerve cell body but also in the surrounding glial cells, some of which divide (Watson, 1974). An early increase in metabolic activity can be detected autoradiographically following the uptake and accumulation of 2-de-

Fig. IV.16. Changes in neuron which are thought to be caused directly or indirectly by loss of a retrograde trophic factor following axotomy.

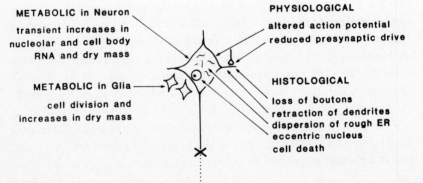

METABOLIC in Neuron

transient increases in
nucleolar and cell body
RNA and dry mass

METABOLIC in Glia

cell division and
increases in dry mass

PHYSIOLOGICAL

altered action potential
reduced presynaptic drive

HISTOLOGICAL

loss of boutons
retraction of dendrites
dispersion of rough ER
eccentric nucleus
cell death

oxyglucose in axotomised neurons (Singer & Mehler, 1980). Physiological techniques show alterations in the action potential waveform recorded in the cell body and a loss of presynaptic drive, which in the electron microscope correlates with the shedding of synaptic boutons, involution of the post-synaptic membrane and retraction of dendrites (e.g. Purves, 1975).

The first attempts to identify the cause of chromatolysis involved detailed observation of the effects of different kinds of nerve injury on motor nerves (Watson, 1974). It was found that the changes were more rapid in onset and more marked when the injury was made closer to the cell body; changes were also more severe when the nerve was cut or ligated, compared with when it was crushed and allowed to reinnervate the distal stump and the target tissue. Suggested causes for these effects include accumulation or depletion of substances normally transported from the cell body, entry of a substance from the circulation at the site of injury, and interruption of a retrograde trophic effect normally exerted on the neurons by the periphery. The latter possibility was favoured by Watson's experiments and other evidence: sensory neurons do not chromatolyse if their central branch in the brain or spinal cord is cut, but they do after damage to the peripheral branch (Carmel & Stein, 1969); moreover, colchicine applied locally to the axons of a variety of neurons produces the same changes as axotomy, presumably by interrupting the flow of a retrograde trophic factor (e.g. Purves, 1976). More recently colchicine applied at low concentration to motor axons blocked retrograde transport (of horseradish peroxidase) *without* producing chromatolysis, and it also *delayed* the increased uptake of 2-deoxyglucose and the histological changes in the cell body produced by cutting the nerve distal to the site of colchicine application (Singer, Mehler & Fernandez, 1982). The interpretation of the effects of colchicine is therefore difficult.

The evidence for a retrograde trophic effect provided by recent experiments on sympathetic and sensory nerves is, however, more convincing. It is now apparent that for these nerves the trophic effect is mediated at least in part by Nerve Growth Factor (NGF). Thus in the adult sympathetic ganglion the effects of post-ganglionic axotomy can be prevented if a pellet releasing NGF is implanted next to the ganglion (Nja & Purves, 1978). More significant is the demonstration that antibodies to NGF produce in the short term some of the changes induced by axotomy, while in the long term (in animals made 'autoimmune' to NGF) the sympathetic neurons atrophy and die (Gorin & Johnson, 1980). Sensory neurons in the same animals do not die but there is a loss of substance P from their central terminals (Schwarz, Pearson & Johnson, 1982), which also occurs after cutting the nerve in the adult (Barbut, Polak & Wall,

1981). The only possible explanation for these effects is that NGF, or an immunologically closely related substance, is present in the normal adult animal and is essential for normal sympathetic and sensory function. Consistent with this explanation is the existence of specific, high-affinity receptors for NGF on the membranes of these neurons, and the fact that NGF taken up by nerve terminals is delivered to the cell body by the fast component of axonal transport (Stockel, Paravicini & Thoenen, 1974). The exact sites of release and uptake of NGF in the animal remain to be determined, but it has been shown that some sympathetically innervated tissues release in culture a substance that is immunologically and biologically indistinguishable from NGF (e.g. Ebendal *et al.*, 1980). Glial cells in culture and degenerating nerve stumps in the animal also release NGF-like material (e.g. Varon, Skaper & Manthorpe, 1981; Lundberg, Longo & Varon, 1982), which suggests that part of the retrograde trophic effect might be mediated via NGF release by glial cells ensheathing the axons.

Much less is known about the agents that mediate the retrograde trophic effects for other kinds of neuron, but it would seem unlikely that adult sympathetic and sensory neurons are unique in their requirement for a factor derived from target or glial cells. More is known about NGF and its trophic effects than about other nerve trophic factors for two important reasons: a simple bioassay for NGF was developed based on the ability of NGF to stimulate axonal outgrowths from ganglia in culture, and a potent source of NGF for experimentation was discovered in the male mouse submaxillary gland (in combination with epidermal growth factor in saliva it assists wound healing: Li *et al.*, 1980). The bioassay techniques have been extended recently to other types of neuron, and factors which promote the survival of these neurons in culture are being isolated from various tissues (see chapter IV.1). One of these factors, a protein required for survival of ciliary ganglion neurons *in vitro*, is released by the ganglion's target tissue and appears to be transported to the cell bodies *in vivo* (Hendry & Hill, 1980). The term 'retrophin' has been coined to describe this, and other similar factors. It is probably only a question of time before these factors are shown to mediate retrograde trophic effects in the adult.

Neurons in invertebrates also show changes suggesting that retrograde trophic influences exist. For example, nerve section or colchicine application to the axon causes insect motor neuron cell bodies, which do not normally generate impulses, to develop a sodium-sensitive action potential (Pitman, 1975). It has also been shown that individual branches of a single lobster motor neuron have very different presynaptic facilitatory characteristics on the different sorts of muscle fibre each branch innervates, suggesting they can be influenced independently by the muscle fibres (Frank, 1973).

Conclusion

Trophic interactions between neurons and their target cells and glia in the adult nervous system operate continuously to maintain the mature innervated state. The trophic effect on muscle is mediated predominantly by post-synaptic activity, but the end-plate region and other post-synaptic cells are probably maintained by a trophic effect of neurotransmitter or other substances released by nerves. Target and glial cells probably maintain their neurons by means of retrograde trophic factors (retrophins).

Interruption of the trophic interactions produces changes in the properties of the cells. Many of the new properties are reminiscent of the embryonic state: target neurons and muscle become supersensitive to transmitter, glia dedifferentiate and axotomised neurons lose their pre-synaptic contacts and dendritic complexity. It is therefore likely that the interactions that occur during development to produce maturation of innervation and target cell properties continue to operate in the adult in the form of the trophic interactions maintaining the mature innervated state. It is also likely that nerve regeneration following injury (see the following chapter) is controlled by some of the mechanisms that first bring about the establishment of innervation.

References

Orthograde trophic effects on peripheral nerve

Droz, B. (1979). How axonal transport contributes to maintenance of the myelin sheath. *Trends in Neurosciences*, **2**, 146–8.

Lubinska, L. (1977). Early course of Wallerian degeneration in myelinated fibres of the rat phrenic nerve. *Brain Research*, **130**, 47–63.

Lubinska, L. (1982). Pattern of Wallerian degeneration of myelinated fibres in short and long peripheral stumps or in isolated segments of rat phrenic nerve. Interpretation of the role of axoplasmic flow of the trophic factor. *Brain Research*, **233**, 227–40.

Miledi, R. & Slater, C.R. (1970). On the degeneration of rat neuromuscular junctions after nerve section. *Journal of Physiology*, **207**, 507–28.

Salzer, J.L. & Bunge, R.P. (1980). Studies of Schwann cell proliferation. I. An analysis in tissue culture of proliferation during development, Wallerian degeneration and direct injury. *Journal of Cell Biology*, **84**, 739–52.

Weinberg, H.J. & Spencer, P.S. (1978). The fate of Schwann cells isolated from axonal contact. *Journal of Neurocytology*, **7**, 555–69.

Orthograde trophic effects on mammalian skeletal muscle

Albuquerque, E.X., Schuh, F.T. & Kauffman, F.C. (1971). Early membrane depolarisation of the fast mammalian muscle after denervation. *Pflügers Archiv für gesamte Physiologie*, **328**, 36–50.

Bray, J.J., Forrest, J.W. & Hubbard, J.I. (1982). Evidence for the role of non-quantal acetylcholine in the maintenance of the membrane potential of rat skeletal muscle. *Journal of Physiology*, **326**, 285–96.

Brown, M.C., Hopkins, W.G. & Keynes, R.J. (1982). Comparison of the effects of denervation and botulinum toxin paralysis on muscle properties in mice. *Journal of Physiology*, **327**, 29–37.

Buller, A.J., Eccles, J.C. & Eccles, R.M. (1960). Interaction between motoneurones and muscles in respect of the characteristic speeds of their responses. *Journal of Physiology*, **150**, 417–39.

Cangiano, A. & Lutzemberger, L. (1980). Partial denervation in inactive muscle affects innervated and denervated fibres equally. *Nature, London*, **285**, 233–5.

Chan-Palay, V., Engel, A.G., Palay, S.C. & Wu, J.-Y. (1982). Synthesizing enzymes for four neuroactive substances in motor neurons and neuromuscular junctions: light and electron microscopic immunocytochemistry. *Proceedings of the National Academy of Sciences, USA*, **79**, 6717–21.

Davey, B., Younkin, L.H. & Younkin, S.G. (1979). Neural control of skeletal muscle cholinesterase: a study using organ-cultured rat muscle. *Journal of Physiology*, **289**, 501–15.

Forrest, J.W., Hills, R.G., Bray, J.J. & Hubbard, J.I. (1981). Calcium-dependent regulation of the membrane potential and extra-junctional acetylcholine receptors of rat skeletal muscle. *Neuroscience*, **6**, 741–9.

Kuromi, H., Gonoi, T. & Hosegawa, S. (1979). Partial purification and characterisation of neurotrophic substance affecting tetrodotoxin sensitivity of organ-cultured mouse muscle. *Brain Research*, **175**, 109–18.

Lømo, T. (1974). Neurotrophic control of colchicine effects on muscle? *Nature, London*, **249**, 473–4.

Lømo, T. & Rosenthal, J. (1972). Control of acetylcholine sensitivity by muscle activity in the rat. *Journal of Physiology*, **221**, 493–513.

Lømo, T., Westgaard, R.H. & Dahl, R.H. (1974). Contractile properties of muscle: control by pattern of muscle activity in the rat. *Proceedings of the Royal Society of London, Series B*, **187**, 99–103.

Salmons, S. & Sreter, F.A. (1976). Significance of impulse activity in the transformation of skeletal muscle types. *Nature, London*, **263**, 30–4.

Weinberg, C.B. & Hall, Z.W. (1979). Junctional form of acetylcholinesterase restored at nerve-free endplates. *Developmental Biology*, **68**, 631–5.

Westgaard, R.H. (1975). Influence of activity on the passive electrical properties of denervated soleus fibres in the rat. *Journal of Physiology*, **251**, 683–97.

Orthograde trophic effects in other tissues

Chalazonitis, A. & Zigmond, R.E. (1980). Effects of synaptic and antidromic stimulation on tyrosine hydroxylase activity in the rat superior cervical ganglion. *Journal of Physiology*, **300**, 425–38.

Dennis, M.J. & Sargent, P.B. (1979). Loss of extrasynaptic ACh sensitivity upon reinnervation of parasympathetic ganglion cells. *Journal of Physiology*, **289**, 263–75.

Frank, E. (1974). The sensitivity to glutamate of denervated muscles of the crayfish. *Journal of Physiology*, **242**, 371–82.

Govind, C.K. & Kent, K.S. (1982). Transformation of fast fibres to slow prevented by lack of activity in developing lobster muscle. *Nature, London*, **298**, 755–7.

Hendry, I.H., Iversen, L.L. & Black, I.B. (1973). A comparison of the neural regulation of tyrosine hydroxylase activity in sympathetic ganglia of adult mice and rats. *Journal of Neurochemistry*, **20**, 1683–9.

Hoy, R.R., Bittner, G.D. & Kennedy, D. (1967). Regeneration in crustacean motoneurons: evidence for axonal fusion. *Science*, **156**, 251–3.

Kuffler, S.W., Dennis, M.J. & Harris, A.J. (1971). The development of chemosensitivity in extra synaptic areas of the neuronal surface after denervation of parasympathetic ganglion cells in the heart of the frog. *Proceedings of the Royal Society of London, Series B*, **177**, 555–63.

Matthews, M.R., Cowan, W.M. & Powell, T.P.S. (1960). Transneuronal cell degeneration in the lateral geniculate nucleus of the macaque monkey. *Journal of Physiology*, **94**, 145–69.

Miledi, R. & Uchitel, O.D. (1981). Induction of action potentials in frog slow muscle fibres paralysed by alpha-bungarotoxin. *Proceedings of the Royal Society of London, Series B*, **213**, 243–8.

Schmidt, H. & Stefani, E. (1977). Action potentials in slow muscle fibres of the frog during regeneration of motor nerves. *Journal of Physiology*, **270**, 507–17.

Singer, M. (1974). Neurotrophic control of limb regeneration in the newt. *Annals of the New York Academy of Sciences, USA*, **228**, 308–22.

Usherwood, P.N.R. (1969). Glutamate sensitivity of denervated insect muscle fibres. *Nature, London*, **223**, 411–13.

Wiesel, T.N. & Hubel, D.H. (1963). Effects of visual deprivation on morphology and physiology of cells in the cat's lateral geniculate body. *Journal of Neurophysiology*, **26**, 978–93.

Zalewski, A.A. (1969). Combined effects of testosterone and motor, sensory or gustatory nerve reinnervation on the regeneration of taste buds. *Experimental Neurology*, **24**, 285–97.

Zigmond, R.E. & Bowers, C.W. (1981). Influence of nerve activity on the macromolecular content of neurons and their effector organs. *Annual Review of Physiology*, **43**, 673–87.

Nerve injury and retrograde trophic effects

Barbut, D., Polak, J. & Wall, P.D. (1981). Substance P in spinal cord dorsal horn decreases following peripheral nerve injury. *Brain Research*, **205**, 289–98.

Carmel, P.W. & Stein, B.M. (1969). Cell changes in sensory ganglia following proximal and distal nerve section in the monkey. *Journal of Comparative Neurology*, **135**, 145–66.

Ebendal, T., Olson, L., Seiger, A. & Hedlund, K.-O. (1980). Nerve growth factors in the rat iris. *Nature, London*, **286**, 25–7.

Frank, E. (1973). Matching of facilitation at the neuromuscular junction of the lobster: a possible case for influence of muscle on nerve. *Journal of Physiology*, **233**, 635–58.

Gorin, P.D. & Johnson, E.M. (1980). Effects of long-term NGF deprivation on the nervous system of the adult rat: an experimental autoimmune approach. *Brain Research*, **198**, 27–42.

Hendry, I.A. & Hill, C.E. (1980). Retrograde axonal transport of target tissue-derived macromolecules. *Nature, London,* **287,** 647–9.

Li, A.K.C., Korody, M.J., Scaltenkerk, M.E., Malt, R.A. & Young, M. (1980). NGF: acceleration of the rate of wound healing in mice. *Proceedings of the National Academy of Sciences, USA,* **77,** 4379–81.

Lundberg, G., Longo, F.M. & Varon, S. (1982). Nerve regeneration model and trophic factors *in vivo. Brain Research,* **232,** 157–61.

Njå, A. & Purves, D. (1978). The effects of nerve growth factor and its antiserum on synapses in the superior cervical ganglion of the guinea pig. *Journal of Physiology,* **277,** 53–75.

Pitman, R.M. (1975). The ionic dependence of action potentials induced by colchicine in an insect motoneurone cell body. *Journal of Physiology,* **247,** 511–20.

Purves, D. (1975). Functional and structural changes in mammalian sympathetic neurones following interruption of their axons. *Journal of Physiology,* **252,** 429–63.

Purves, D. (1976). Functional and structural changes in mammalian sympathetic neurones following colchicine application to post-ganglionic nerves. *Journal of Physiology,* **259,** 159–75.

Schwarz, J.P., Pearson, J. & Johnson, E.M. (1982). Effects of exposure to anti-NGF on sensory neurons of adult rats and guinea pigs. *Brain Research,* **244,** 378–81.

Singer, P.A. & Mehler, S. (1980). 2-Deoxy[^{14}C]glucose uptake in rat hypoglossal nucleus after nerve transection. *Experimental Neurology,* **69,** 617–26.

Singer, P.A., Mehler, S. & Fernandez, H.L. (1982). Blockade of retrograde axonal transport delays the onset of metabolic and morphological changes induced by axotomy. *Journal of Neuroscience,* **2,** 1299–306.

Stockel, K., Paravicini, U. & Thoenen, H. (1974). Specificity of the retrograde axonal transport of nerve growth factor. *Brain Research,* **76,** 413–21.

Varon, S., Skaper, S.D. & Manthorpe, M. (1981). Trophic activities for dorsal root and sympathetic ganglionic neurons in media conditioned by Schwann and other peripheral cells. *Developmental Brain Research,* **1,** 73–87.

Watson, W.E. (1974). Cellular responses to axotomy and to related procedures. *British Medical Bulletin,* **30,** 112–15.

IV.5

Nerve growth and synaptic modifications induced by injury

Introduction

Nerve injury in the adult usually elicits new nerve outgrowths which can reinnervate and restore function to denervated target tissues. In the peripheral nervous system of nearly all species and the CNS of many lower forms, damage to a nerve produces regeneration of the axons from the proximal stump, and the new outgrowths can be guided back to their original target cells by the structures in the degenerating distal nerve segment (fig. IV.17). Such regeneration is uncommon in the CNS of mammals, but here and in the peripheral nervous system intact axons in any partly denervated target can also develop new outgrowths called collateral sprouts, which reinnervate the vacated post-synaptic sites (fig. IV.17). Nerve regeneration and nerve sprouting both appear to be controlled predominantly at the site of new growth, probably by factors which stimulate growth and surfaces which guide or permit growth. The nerve cell body may also play a role by limiting the extent of new growth and switching to a metabolic state appropriate for growth.

Nerve injury can also lead to the 'unmasking' of synapses that are functionally ineffective in the normal animal. In some cases tonic activity in a pathway appears to repress the synapses, which are disinhibited as soon as activity is interrupted by injury. In other cases unmasking develops more slowly as cells react to the injury.

Axonal regeneration

Regrowth from the proximal stump of an axon begins 1–2 days after the lesion in mammalian peripheral nerves, and growth rates of the order of a few millimetres per day are possible. If the lesion is a nerve crush, each regenerating axon remains within the basement membrane and collagenous sheath that originally enclosed the intact axon and its Schwann cells. Complete reinnervation is therefore usual because the axons are guided back to their original target cells. When a nerve is cut and the cut ends are sutured together many of the axons regenerate down inappropriate sheaths and the resulting restoration of function is less complete. If the cut ends are not sutured together glial cells dividing and migrating out from the ends may produce a bridge between the proximal and distal stumps, and axons growing out on these glial cells may still be able to enter the distal stump and hence reach the target tissues. In mammals failure of axons to find the distal stump produces a tangled mass of nervous tissue called a neuroma, but in lower vertebrates axons are capable of continued growth through adjacent tissues and can finally reach and reinnervate their specific targets (for references see Sunderland, 1978).

Fig. IV.17. Nerve growth induced by injury in the adult. Axon regeneration and collateral sprouting are shown here for motor axons following a crush injury of a spinal nerve. Note that nodal sprouts only arise from nodes *within* the muscle, usually from nodes near to end-plates.

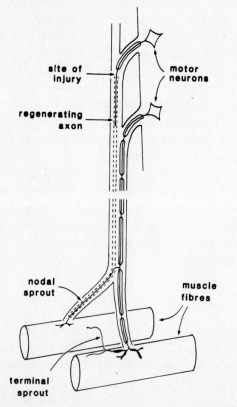

It was established by Lubinska (1952) that regeneration in the first few days following crush injury is delayed until degenerative changes in the denervated peripheral nerve progress to a certain stage. One of the changes is likely to be simply a physical clearing of the axonal pathway to permit access by the regenerating axon. There could also be changes in the surface membranes or basement membranes of the glial cells, and there is now considerable evidence that the production by the glial cells of growth factors is important. Glial cells *in vitro* and *in vivo* have been shown to produce growth factors (Varon, Skaper & Manthorpe, 1981; Lundberg, Longo & Varon, 1982). Moreover, Nerve Growth Factor (NGF) is probably involved in the regeneration of peripheral adrenergic axons and axons of the retinal ganglion cells in the optic nerve, since regeneration of these axons is enhanced by injections of NGF and inhibited by injections of antiserum to NGF (Bjerre, Bjorklund & Edwards, 1974; Turner & Glaze, 1977; Glaze & Turner, 1978). It is not yet known whether other growth factors are involved in the regeneration of other types of nerve, but extracts from rat hippocampus can stimulate growth of chick ciliary and sympathetic ganglia grown in culture. The growth of the latter cells is due to NGF in the extract but another agent (as yet unidentified) is responsible for the parasympathetic stimulation (Crutcher & Collins, 1982).

Regeneration also appears to be under the control of the cell body to some extent. This has been shown with an experimental paradigm in which growth elicited by a test lesion is compared with that when the nerve has been previously primed with a conditioning lesion made at a more distal site. In peripheral sensory and motor nerves a conditioning lesion produces a significant enhancement of growth (e.g. McQuarrie, 1978), so it is likely that a change which enhances regeneration gradually develops in the neuron in the days following injury. Oddly, regeneration of peripheral adrenergic neurons is inhibited by a conditioning lesion (McQuarrie *et al.*, 1978). Regeneration of the optic nerve in fish and amphibians is also enhanced by a conditioning injury, and if the retina is excised and cultured in the presence of NGF the development of axonal outgrowths is markedly advanced and enhanced by a prior lesion to the optic nerve (Turner, Schwab & Thoenen, 1982). It appears, therefore, that the retinal ganglion cell axons develop increased responsiveness to NGF following injury. Whether this applies to all types of injured axon remains to be seen.

It is unfortunate for many accident victims that most axons in the CNS regenerate poorly following injury. The most likely reason for this is the absence in the CNS of the robust endoneurial sheaths that guide regenerating axons in the periphery. Central neurons will invade and grow vigorously along such sheaths if a segment of peripheral nerve is inserted into the brain (Richardson, McGuiness & Aguayo, 1980). Scar tissue formation at the site of injury may be another factor contributing to poor central regeneration: destruction of monoaminergic axons without disturbance to surrounding tissues can be produced by chemical axotomy with neurotoxins such as 6-hydroxydopamine, and following such treatments the axons regenerate quite successfully (e.g. Nobin *et al.*, 1973). Finally adult central neurons may be partly responsible for their own poor regeneration, because embryonic monoaminergic and cholinergic neurons transplanted to adult brains to replace corresponding lesioned nuclei can reinnervate the denervated target neurons and restore function (e.g. Low *et al.*, 1982).

Collateral sprouting

Intact axons, not directly involved in damage, can respond to the denervation of neighbouring territory by developing new outgrowths (collateral sprouts) which innervate the denervated neurons or tissue. This was first suspected at the turn of the century when it was found that partly denervated muscles recovered their strength quickly and contained few atrophied muscle fibres, even before the cut axons had regenerated. Similar functional recovery following partial denervation in the peripheral nervous system has been demonstrated in some skin sensory nerves (e.g. Devor *et al.*, 1979) and in autonomic ganglia (Murray & Thompson, 1957; Courtney & Roper, 1976). In the 1950s histological investigations of partly denervated muscles and ganglia stained with silver confirmed that the denervated target cells had become reinnervated by outgrowths from the remaining intact axons.

Sprouting in the CNS was first detected indirectly following transection of all but one dorsal root on one side of the spinal cord. Weeks later sprouting of the branches of the intact root in the cord was inferred when this root and its partner on the contralateral control side were cut in order to produce acute degeneration, which could be detected by a silver stain. More widespread degeneration was found on the experimental side and hence it was concluded that sprouting had occurred (Liu & Chambers, 1958). Direct visualisation of the branches of the intact afferents with horseradish peroxidase has failed to confirm the occurrence of sprouting in this experiment (Rodin *et al.*, 1983) but it is nevertheless clear that injury-induced sprouting does occur at many other CNS loci. The direct histological methods used to detect the sprouting include axon stains, axon tracers, stains specific for transmitter and transmitter enzymes, and electron microscopy to visualise synapses produced by the sprouts (e.g. Raisman & Field, 1973). Electrophysiological recording has shown that at least some of these synapses can transmit (e.g. Lynch, Deadwyler & Cotman, 1973), and in several studies behavioural assay has revealed that the loss of function produced by a nerve lesion is partly restored following sprouting (e.g. Goldberger, 1977; Loesche & Steward, 1977). Sprouting may therefore help to account for recovery following brain damage.

Sprouting in the CNS of developing animals is vigorous and the sprouts can travel long distances (e.g. Tsukahara, 1981). Sprouting in the CNS of adults is in contrast much less pronounced: many nerves do not sprout and the sprouts of those that do probably remain localised to the dendrites which have been deafferented (see review by Cotman, Nieto-Sampedro & Harris, 1981). Presumably the same factors that limit regeneration in the CNS also limit sprouting.

The nature of the stimulus for sprouting has been investigated predominantly in muscle, where it is possible to distinguish new outgrowths arising either from nodes of Ranvier (*nodal sprouts*) or from intact nerve terminals (*terminal sprouts*) (see fig. IV.17, and review by Brown, Holland & Hopkins, 1981). In the 1950s it was thought that terminal and nodal sprouting might be stimulated by the release of some abnormal agent from degenerating nerves or myelin. Indeed, lipid extracts of nerve and other tissues were found to stimulate sprouting. However, terminal sprouting is observed without degeneration when muscles are rendered inactive by various means (e.g. Duchen & Strich, 1968; Brown & Ironton, 1977), and terminal sprouting is inhibited if partly denervated or inactive muscle fibres are electrically stimulated (Ironton, Brown & Holland, 1978). This implies that it is the muscle fibres that produce the terminal sprouting stimulus when they become inactive following denervation. Nerve degeneration products or lipid extracts probably stimulate terminal sprouting indirectly by causing an 'inflammatory effect' which produces denervation-like changes in muscle fibres, including presumably increased production of a sprouting stimulus (Brown, Holland & Ironton, 1978).

The terminal sprouting stimulus appears to be able to diffuse to intact nerve terminals from inactive (Betz, Caldwell & Ribchester, 1980) or denervated (Brown & Holland, 1979) muscle fibres within a muscle, yet it seems unable to reach further than to an immediately adjacent fibre (Brown, Holland, Hopkins & Keynes, 1980; Slack & Pockett, 1981). This limited range of diffusion is difficult to explain if the growth stimulus is a protein like NGF, and it raises the possibility that nerve terminal growth is controlled by surface changes on muscle fibres. The stimulus may be, for example, a component of the basement membrane of denervated muscle fibres which stimulates growth by providing a suitable substrate for attachment of terminal outgrowths. Alternatively, there may be need for a surface change *and* a diffusible growth factor before sprouts can form and then grow.

Nodal sprouting (fig. IV.17) differs from terminal sprouting in several important respects. The nodal sprouting response to partial denervation is not inhibited by direct muscle stimulation (Ironton *et al.*, 1978), nor is it enhanced by a conditioning period of muscle paralysis prior to partial denervation (Brown, Hopkins & Keynes, 1982). The suggestion that nodal sprouting is controlled by a requirement for sufficient dedifferentiation of the Schwann cell pathways to permit sprout growth to denervated end-plates finds some support in the pattern of nodal sprout growth (Hopkins & Slack, 1981) and the pattern of degeneration of the denervated pathways (Brown *et al.*, 1982). Nevertheless a factor from muscle may still be involved, perhaps in initiating nodal sprout growth. Thus some atypical nodal sprouts are observed in paralysed muscles without nerve degeneration (Hopkins, Brown & Keynes, 1981), and selective destruction of the end-plate region of muscle fibres at the time of partial denervation inhibits subsequent nodal sprouting (Keynes, Hopkins & Brown, 1982). One possible explanation for all these observations is that the nodal sprouting stimulus is released from the end-plate and that its release from this site is not inhibited by muscle stimulation. The same stimulus released from the extrajunctional membrane of inactive muscle fibres may also help to evoke terminal and nodal sprouting.

A role for a target-released factor in sprouting has also been suggested by observation of the effect of the drug colchicine on nerve growth. A critical dose of colchicine applied locally to nerves can block axonal transport without initially causing degeneration. If it is applied to one of the nerves innervating the skin of axolotls the receptive field of an adjoining nerve expands into the territory of the blocked nerve (Cooper, Diamond & Turner, 1977). It has been suggested that colchicine blocks an orthograde nerve trophic effect on the sensory end-organs, which then produce a nerve growth stimulus to which unblocked nerves respond. A detailed histological study of the nerve plexuses in the skin might give some clue as to whether this or some other change induced by colchicine underlies the induced sprouting. Colchicine-induced blockade of transport in some afferents to the hippocampus also stimulates growth, presumably in the unblocked afferents, and a similar mechanism may be involved (Goldowitz & Cotman, 1980). In addition colchicine stimulates immediate growth in nerve terminals when it is applied to frog motor nerves, although it is less clear how this effect might be mediated (Rotshenker, 1981).

The nerve cell body does not appear to be involved in sprouting directly. For example, even if there is a metabolic change in the neuron induced by a peripheral stimulus, the sprouting is still localised to axonal branches in the regions producing the stimulus (Slack & Pockett, 1981). However, effects on the cell body *can* be manifest in sprouting in the periphery, as has been demonstrated in experiments by Rotshenker (1979). He has shown that denervating a frog muscle produces sprouting in the contralateral muscle, and he hypothesises that some signal for growth spreads from the axotomised and regenerating motor neurons across the spinal cord. However, this phenomenon does not occur in mice (Brown, Holland & Ironton, 1980). Finally the ability of the cell body to establish or maintain sprouts probably sets the limit on the amount of sprouting that can be produced in response to growth stimuli from the periphery. Motor units, for example, can expand to no more than five times their normal size (Brown & Ironton, 1978). ·

These observations on sprouting indicate that it is a local growth response to a stimulus produced locally in a target tissue. At present it is not certain how the local stimulus to sprouting is related to events during development, but it is likely that sprouting is triggered by release from the denervated adult tissue of the same growth factor for which neurons and their branches are thought to compete in embryogenesis and early post-natal life. The recent finding that the end-plate region of denervated muscle contains a motor neuron survival factor is consistent with this view (Slack & Pockett, 1982).

Unmasking of suppressed synapses

The concept of structurally normal but functionally inactive synapses was first raised to prominence following experiments on the reinnervation of denervated eye muscles in fish (Mark, 1970). The results of the experiments suggested that the terminals of a foreign nerve that had innervated the muscles were not withdrawn when the correct nerve regenerated; instead it appeared that they remained on the fibres as 'silent' synapses that could be quickly reactivated or 'unmasked' if the correct nerve was cut a second time. Although more careful investigation showed that functionally suppressed synapses were not present in either the fish eye muscles (Scott, 1975) or in comparable reinnervated amphibian muscles (Dennis & Yip, 1978), there is nevertheless now considerable evidence for the existence of such synapses in the CNS.

Examples of rapidly induced changes in the visual system that can be attributed to derepression of suppressed synapses in the visual cortex have been discussed already in chapter IV.2 (p. 83). Wall and his colleagues, in their studies of receptive fields of neurons in the somatosensory pathway, have provided evidence that the phenomenon occurs also in the spinal cord. Cells in the dorsal column nuclei (a sensory relay in the spinal cord) develop novel receptive fields as soon as their normal inputs are cut in the dorsal roots or blocked by local cooling in the cord (Dostrovsky, Millar & Wall, 1976). The fact that these changes occur so quickly implies that the new receptive fields arise from pre-existing suppressed synapses which are derepressed when some inhibitory effect resulting from tonic activity in the sensory axons is interrupted. Subliminal inputs can also be revealed by strong electrical stimulation of sensory nerves (Dostrovsky, Jabbur & Millar, 1978), and immediate changes in receptive fields occur if the level of excitability of cells and presynaptic terminals in the dorsal column is increased by infusion of 4-aminopyridine (Saade *et al.*, 1982).

New receptive fields also develop over a period of days to weeks in cells in the thalamus following lesions of their normal inputs from dorsal column nuclei, and in cells in the dorsal column nuclei and dorsal horn of the cord following section of dorsal roots. Indirect evidence suggests that unmasking of existing synapses could account for these new receptive fields, but the delay in their appearance and the presence of nerve degeneration mean that sprouting cannot be ruled out (Merrill & Wall, 1978).

Section of a peripheral sensory nerve in rats also produces within a week new receptive fields on dorsal horn cells that are normally driven only by the sectioned nerve (Devor & Wall, 1981; fig. IV.18), and in this case the evidence strongly favours unmasking. Sprouting of the intact afferents could not be detected with a stain specific for some sensory nerve terminals in the cord (Devor & Claman, 1980) and degeneration of the terminals of the injured nerve on the dorsal horn cells could not be detected within 10 days of injury. An early decrease in the dorsal root potential in the roots of the damaged nerve paralleled the development of the new receptive fields, so it is likely that decreased presynaptic inhibition from the surround is responsible for unmasking the synapses (Wall & Devor, 1981). Substance P

Fig. IV.18. Unmasking of synapses on dorsal horn neurons following peripheral nerve cut.

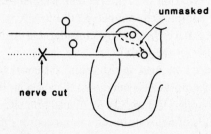

could be the neurotransmitter mediating this inhibition because there is an early loss of substance P from sensory terminals following a cut injury (Barbut, Polak & Wall, 1981). The signal for unmasking may be associated with the uptake by the nerve of some substance from the circulation, because the new receptive fields do not develop if the peripheral nerve is crushed rather than cut (Devor & Wall, 1981), but it is also possible that unmasking is associated with the metabolic changes that accompany interruption of a retrograde trophic factor, probably NGF.

The significance of suppressed synapses is still a matter for conjecture. They are probably a remnant from the period of diffuse innervation in the neonate, but whether they help maintain sensation following peripheral nerve injury, or whether at higher levels they play a part in learning and memory, is less clear.

References

Axonal regeneration

Bjerre, B., Bjorklund, A. & Edwards, D.C. (1974). Axonal regeneration of peripheral adrenergic neurons: effects of antiserum to NGF in mouse. *Cell and Tissue Research*, **148**, 441–76.

Crutcher, K.A. & Collins, F. (1982). *In vitro* evidence for two distinct hippocampal growth factors: basis for neuronal plasticity? *Science*, **217**, 67–8.

Glaze, K.A. & Turner, J.E. (1978). Regenerative repair in the severed optic nerve of the newt (*Triturus viridescens*): effect of nerve growth factor antiserum. *Experimental Neurology*, **58**, 500–10.

Low, W.C., Lewis, P.R., Bunch, S.T., Dunnett, S.B., Thomas, S.R., Iversen, S.D., Bjorklund, A. & Stenevi, U. (1982). Function recovery following neural transplantation of embryonic septal nuclei in adult rats with septohippocampal lesions. *Nature, London*, **300**, 260–2.

Lubinska, L. (1952). The influence of the state of the peripheral stump on the early stages of nerve regeneration. *Acta biologica experimentalis, Warsaw*, **16**, 55–63.

Lundberg, G., Longo, F.M. & Varon, S. (1982). Nerve regeneration model and trophic factors *in vivo*. *Brain Research*, **232**, 157–61.

McQuarrie, I.G. (1978). The effect of a conditioning lesion on the regeneration of motor axons. *Brain Research*, **152**, 597–602.

McQuarrie, I.G., Grafstein, B., Dreyfus, B.C.F. & Gershon, M.B. (1978). Regeneration of adrenergic axons in rat sciatic nerve: effect of a conditioning lesion. *Brain Research*, **141**, 21–34.

Nobin, A., Baumgarten, H.G., Bjorklund, A., Lachenmayer, L. & Stenevi, U. (1973). Axonal degeneration and regeneration of the bulbospinal indolamine neurons after 5,6-dihydroxytryptamine treatment. *Brain Research*, **56**, 1–24.

Richardson, P.M., McGuiness, U.M. & Aguayo, A.J. (1980). Axons from CNS neurones regenerate into PNS grafts. *Nature, London*, **284**, 264–5.

Sunderland, S. (1978). *Nerves and Nerve Injuries*, 2nd edn. London: Churchill Livingstone.

Turner, J.E. & Glaze, K.A. (1977). Regenerative repair in the severed optic nerve of the newt (*Triturus viridescens*): effect of nerve growth factor. *Experimental Neurology*, **57**, 687–97.

Turner, J.E., Schwab, M.E. & Thoenen, M. (1982). NGF stimulates neurite outgrowth from goldfish retinal explants: the influence of a prior lesion. *Developmental Brain Research*, **4**, 59–86.

Varon, S., Skaper, S.D. & Manthorpe, M. (1981). Trophic activities for dorsal root and sympathetic ganglionic neurons in media conditioned by Schwann and other peripheral cells. *Developmental Brain Research*, **1**, 73–87.

Collateral sprouting

Betz, W.J., Caldwell, J.H. & Ribchester, R.R. (1980). Sprouting of active nerve terminals in partially inactive muscles of the rat. *Journal of Physiology*, **303**, 281–97.

Brown, M.C. & Holland, R.L. (1979). A central role for denervated tissues in causing nerve sprouting. *Nature, London*, **282**, 724–6.

Brown, M.C., Holland, R.L. & Hopkins, W.G. (1981). Motor nerve sprouting. *Annual Review of Neuroscience*, **4**, 17–42.

Brown, M.C., Holland, R.L., Hopkins, W.G. & Keynes, R.J. (1980). An assessment of the spread of the signal for terminal sprouting within and between muscles. *Brain Research*, **210**, 145–51.

Brown, M.C., Holland, R.L. & Ironton, R. (1978). Degenerating nerve products affect innervated muscle fibres. *Nature, London*, **275**, 652–4.

Brown, M.C., Holland, R.L. & Ironton, R. (1980). Nodal and terminal sprouting from motor nerves in fast and slow muscles of the mouse. *Journal of Physiology*, **306**, 493–510.

Brown, M.C., Hopkins, W.G. & Keynes, R.J. (1982). Importance of pathway formation for nodal sprout production in partly denervated muscles. *Brain Research*, **243**, 345–9.

Brown, M.C. & Ironton, R. (1977). Motor neurone sprouting induced by prolonged tetrodotoxin block of nerve action potentials. *Nature, London*, **265**, 459–61.

Brown, M.C. & Ironton, R. (1978). Sprouting and regression of neuromuscular synapses in partially denervated mammalian muscles. *Journal of Physiology*, **278**, 325–8.

Cooper, E., Diamond, J. & Turner, C. (1977). The effects of nerve section and of colchicine treatment on the density of mechanosensory nerve endings in salamander skin. *Journal of Physiology*, **264**, 725–49.

Cotman, C.W., Nieto-Sampedro, M. & Harris, E.W. (1981). Synapse replacement in the nervous system of adult vertebrates. *Physiological Reviews*, **61**, 684–784.

Courtney, K. & Roper, S. (1976). Sprouting of synapses after partial denervation of frog cardiac ganglion. *Nature, London*, **259**, 317–19.

Devor, M. & Claman, D. (1980). Mapping and plasticity of acid phosphatase afferents in the rat dorsal horn. *Brain Research*, **190**, 17–28.

Devor, M., Schonfeld, D., Seltzer, Z. & Wall, P.D. (1979). Two modes of cutaneous reinnervation following peripheral nerve injury. *Journal of Comparative Neurology*, **185**, 211–20.

Devor, M. & Wall, P.D. (1981). Plasticity in the spinal cord sensory map following peripheral nerve injury. *Journal of Neuroscience*, **1**, 679–84.

Duchen, L. & Strich, S. (1968). The effects of botulinum toxin on the pattern of innervation of skeletal muscle of the mouse. *Quarterly Journal of Experimental Physiology*, **53**, 84–9.

Goldberger, M.E. (1977). Locomotor recovery after unilateral hindlimb deafferentation. *Brain Research*, **123**, 59–74.

Goldowitz, D. & Cotman, C.W. (1980). Do neurotrophic interactions control synapse formation in the adult rat brain? *Brain Research*, **181**, 325–44.

Hopkins, W.G., Brown, M.C. & Keynes, R.J. (1981). Nerve growth from nodes of Ranvier in inactive muscle. *Brain Research*, **222**, 125–8.

Hopkins, W.G. & Slack, J.R. (1981). The sequential development of nodal sprouts in mouse muscles in response to nerve degeneration. *Journal of Neurocytology*, **10**, 537–56.

Ironton, R., Brown, M.C. & Holland, R.L. (1978). Stimuli to intramuscular nerve growth. *Brain Research*, **156**, 351–4.

Keynes, R.J., Hopkins, W.G. & Brown, M.C. (1982). Sprouting of mammalian motor neurones at nodes of Ranvier: the role of the denervated motor endplate. *Brain Research*, **264**, 209–13.

Liu, C.-M. & Chambers, W.W. (1958). Intraspinal sprouting of dorsal root axons. *Archives of Neurology and Psychiatry*, **79**, 46–61.

Loesche, J. & Steward, D. (1977). Behavioural correlates of denervation and reinnervation of the hippocampal formation of the rat: recovery of alternation performance following unilateral entorhinal cortex lesions. *Brain Research Bulletin*, **2**, 21–39.

Lynch, G., Deadwyler, S. & Cotman, C.W. (1973). Postlesion axonal growth produces permanent functional connections. *Science*, **180**, 1364–6.

Murray, J.G. & Thompson, J.W. (1957). The occurrence and function of collateral sprouting in the sympathetic nervous system of the cat. *Journal of Physiology*, **135**, 133–62.

Raisman, G. & Field, P.M. (1973). A quantitative investigation of the development of collateral reinnervation after partial deafferentation of the septal nuclei. *Brain Research*, **50**, 241–64.

Rodin, B.E., Sampogna, S.L. & Kruger, L. (1983). An examination of intraspinal sprouting in dorsal root axons with the tracer HRP. *Journal of Comparative Neurology*, **215**, 187–98.

Rotshenker, S. (1979). Synapse formation in intact innervated cutaneous pectoris muscles of the frog following denervation of the opposite muscle. *Journal of Physiology*, **292**, 535–47.

Rotshenker, S. (1981). Sprouting and synapse formation by motor axons separated from their cell bodies. *Brain Research*, **223**, 141–5.

Slack, J.R. & Pockett, S. (1981). Terminal sprouting is a local response to a local stimulus. *Brain Research*, **217**, 368–74.

Slack, J.R. & Pockett, S. (1982). Motor neurotrophic factor in adult skeletal muscle. *Brain Research*, **247**, 138–40.

Tsukahara, N. (1981). Sprouting and the neuronal basis of learning. *Trends in Neurosciences*, **4**, 234–7.

Unmasking of suppressed synapses

Barbut, D., Polak, J. & Wall, P.D. (1981). Substance P in spinal cord dorsal horn decreases following peripheral nerve injury. *Brain Research*, **205**, 289–98.

Dennis, M.J. & Yip, J.W. (1978). Formation and elimination of foreign synapses on adult salamander muscle. *Journal of Physiology*, **274**, 299–310.

Devor, M. & Claman, D. (1980). Mapping and plasticity of acid phosphatase afferents in the rat dorsal horn. *Brain Research*, **190**, 17–28.

Devor, M. & Wall, P.D. (1981). Plasticity in the spinal cord sensory map following peripheral nerve injury in rats. *Journal of Neuroscience*, **1**, 679–84.

Dostrovsky, J.O., Jabbur, S. & Millar, J. (1978). Neurons in cat gracile nucleus with both local and widefield inputs. *Journal of Physiology*, **278**, 365–75.

Dostrovsky, J.O., Millar, J. & Wall, P.D. (1976). The immediate shift of afferent drive of dorsal column nucleus cells following deafferentation: a comparison of acute and chronic deafferentation in gracile nucleus and spinal cord. *Experimental Neurology*, **52**, 480–95.

Mark, R.F. (1970). Chemospecific synaptic repression as a possible memory store. *Nature, London*, **225**, 178–9.

Merrill, E.G. & Wall, P.D. (1978). Plasticity of connections in the adult nervous system. In *Neuronal Plasticity*, ed. C.W. Cotman, pp. 97–112. New York: Raven Press.

Saade, N.E., Banna, N.R., Khoury, A., Jabbur, S.J. & Wall, P.D. (1982). Cutaneous receptive field alterations induced by 4-aminopyridine. *Brain Research*, **232**, 177–80.

Scott, S.A. (1975). Persistence of foreign innervation on reinnervated goldfish extraocular muscles. *Science*, **189**, 644–6.

Wall, P.D. & Devor, M. (1981). The effect of peripheral nerve injury on dorsal root potentials and on transmission of afferent signals into the spinal cord. *Brain Research*, **209**, 95–111.

Conclusion to part IV

Two major themes have emerged in this part of the book on modification of connections. The first is the dependence of pre- and post-synaptic elements on each other's presence. This dependence demands that during development neurons make and receive adequate connections, and failure to do so probably accounts for neuronal death and elimination and redistribution of synapses. In the adult the mutual interdependence of neurons is revealed by the changes in properties of pre- and post-synaptic neurons whenever communications between them are interrupted.

A start has only just been made on discovering the factors which mediate the interdependence of neurons. In the retrograde direction there is evidence that specific molecules manufactured by the target cell or neuron are taken up at synaptic sites and transported retrogradely to the soma. The most well characterised of these substances is Nerve Growth Factor, which is a 'retrophin' for post-ganglionic sympathetic and sensory neurons in mammals. Other retrophins are now being isolated. In the orthograde direction, substances released by nerves influence glia and target cell properties. For muscle the substance is the neurotransmitter, which exerts its effects predominantly via the action potentials it elicits, but at the end-plate and at other targets the transmitter probably has effects independent of action potentials.

A speculative scheme summarising the way in which orthograde and retrograde trophic effects may interact during development is shown in fig. IV.19. With the onset of innervation orthograde trophic effects begin to operate. This may reduce the supply of retrograde trophic substances, leading first to neuronal death and then to elimination of some axonal branches. The state of the adult tissues is not fixed permanently following these developmental interactions, but is maintained by the continuing interaction of pre- and post-synaptic elements. A decreased supply of retrophin to the cell body following axotomy may be responsible for various changes in the cell body and in central connections, and an increased production of retrophin by denervated target tissue may be responsible for collateral sprouting.

The importance of synchronous activity in shaping neuronal connections is the other theme in part IV. Synchrony of activity in the pre- and post-synaptic elements of a synapse appears to increase the probability of survival of the synapse during the period when excess connections are eliminated. In the visual system synchrony is in part responsible for establishing the characteristic patterns of banding of afferents and the fine-tuning of receptive fields. Elsewhere in the nervous system it may mediate in the functional validation of axon branches and possibly also in the competitive interaction at the neuromuscular junction. The way in which synchrony achieves its effects on these axonal connections is still unclear, but it could involve stabilisation of receptors or the release and uptake of retrophin.

Synchronous activity in two convergent inputs resulting in permanent changes in synaptic effectiveness of one of them, has been identified as the basis of learning at several sites in the nervous system. In the invertebrate *Aplysia* the changes in the synapse are brought about by a presynaptic mechanism, while in the mammalian cerebellum post-synaptic receptors appear to be altered. Long-term potentiation of synaptic transmission by trains of activity may be associated with the acquisition of memory in the hippocampus, and this appears to involve pre- and post-synaptic changes. Other modifications that may be the basis of learning and memory at these and other sites in the nervous system have yet to be determined.

Fig. IV.19. The inverse relationship that may exist between levels of orthograde and retrograde trophic effects as connections are established and modified.

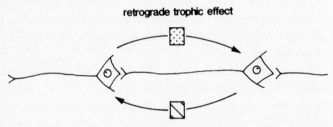

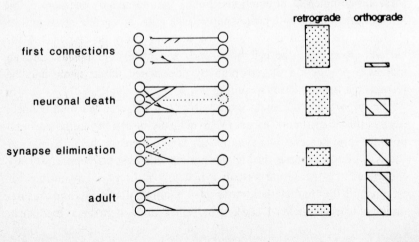

Index